MILADY STANDARD COSMETOLOGY

Practical
Workbook

MILADY STANDARD COSMETOLOGY

Practical Workbook

To be used with

Milady Standard Cosmetology

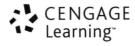
CENGAGE
Learning™

Australia • Brazil • Japan • Korea • Mexico • Singapore • Spain • United Kingdom • United States

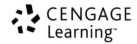

**Milady Standard Cosmetology
Practical Workbook**
Lisha Barnes

President, Milady: Dawn Gerrain

Associate Acquisitions Editor: Philip Mandl

Editorial Assistant: Maria K. Hebert

Director of Beauty Industry Relations:
Sandra Bruce

Executive Marketing Manager: Gerard McAvey

Production Director: Wendy Troeger

Senior Content Project Manager:
Angela Sheehan

Art Director: Benj Gleeksman

Cover Image: © Adrianna Williams/Corbis

For product information and technology assistance, contact us at
Professional & Career Group Customer Support, 1-800-648-7450

For permission to use material from this text or product,
submit all requests online at **www.cengage.com/permissions**
Further permissions questions can be emailed to
permissionrequest@cengage.com

Library of Congress Control Number: 2010903896

ISBN-13: 978-1-4390-5922-7

ISBN-10: 1-4390-5922-5

Milady
5 Maxwell Drive
Clifton Park, NY 12065-2919
USA

Cengage Learning products are represented in Canada by Nelson Education, Ltd.

For your course and learning solutions, visit **milady.cengage.com**

Visit our corporate Web site at **cengage.com.**

Notice to the Reader
Publisher does not warrant or guarantee any of the products described herein or perform any independent analysis in connection with any of the product information contained herein. Publisher does not assume, and expressly disclaims, any obligation to obtain and include information other than that provided to it by the manufacturer. The reader is expressly warned to consider and adopt all safety precautions that might be indicated by the activities described herein and to avoid all potential hazards. By following the instructions contained herein, the reader willingly assumes all risks in connection with such instructions. The publisher makes no representations or warranties of any kind, including but not limited to, the warranties of fitness for particular purpose or merchantability, nor are any such representations implied with respect to the material set forth herein, and the publisher takes no responsibility with respect to such material. The publisher shall not be liable for any special, consequential, or exemplary damages resulting, in whole or part, from the readers' use of, or reliance upon, this material.

Printed in the United States of America
3 4 5 6 7 15 14 13 12

Contents

How to Use this Workbook

Milady Standard Cosmetology Practical Workbook has been written to meet the needs, interests, and abilities of students receiving training in cosmetology.

This workbook should be used together with *Milady Standard Cosmetology* and *Milady Standard Cosmetology Theory Workbook.* This book directly follows the practical information found in the student textbook. Pages to be read and studied are listed at the beginning of each chapter. The theory information can be found in *Milady Standard Cosmetology Theory Workbook.*

Students are to answer each item in this workbook with a pencil after consulting their textbook for correct information. Items can be corrected and/or rated during class or individual discussions, or on an independent study basis.

Various tests are included to emphasize essential facts found in the textbook and to measure the student's progress.

CHAPTER 1 History and Career Opportunities

See Milady Standard Cosmetology Theory Workbook.

CHAPTER 2 Life Skills

See Milady Standard Cosmetology Theory Workbook.

CHAPTER 3 Your Professional Image

See Milady Standard Cosmetology Theory Workbook.

CHAPTER 4 Communicating for Success

See Milady Standard Cosmetology Theory Workbook.

5 Infection Control: Principles and Practices

Date: _____

Rating: _____

Text Pages: 65–107

POINT TO PONDER:

"Every worthwhile accomplishment has a price tag attached to it. The question is always whether you are willing to pay the price to attain it—in hard work, sacrifice, patience, faith, and endurance."—**John C. Maxwell**

WHY STUDY INFECTION CONTROL: PRINCIPLES AND PRACTICES?

1. List the three main reasons why it is important for cosmetologists to study and thoroughly understand infection control principles and practices.

a) _____

_____

_____

b) _____

_____

_____

c) _____

_____

_____

REGULATION

2. State agencies set guidelines for the manufacturing, sale, and use of equipment and chemical ingredients.

_____ True

_____ False

3. OSHA is part of the U.S. Department of _____.

4. The _____ created the Hazard Communication Standard (HCS), which requires that chemical manufacturers and importers assess the potential hazards associated with their products.

5. The standards set by OSHA address which of the following issues?

_____ a) Handling and mixing of products

_____ b) General workplace safety

_____ c) Potentially hazardous product ingredients

_____ d) All of these answers are correct.

6. _____ laws require that manufacturers supply a Material Safety Data Sheet (MSDS) for all products sold.

_____ a) Federal

_____ b) State

_____ c) Both a and b are correct.

_____ d) Neither a nor b is correct.

7. Where should you look to locate the names of hazardous ingredients used in a chemical salon product?

_____ a) The manufacturer's invoice

_____ b) The product's MSDS

_____ c) The salon's employee handbook

_____ d) The EPA's website

8. How does an employee verify that he or she has read an MSDS?

_____

_____

9. Disinfectants are used to destroy all BUT which of the following?

_____ a) Bacteria

_____ b) Fungi

_____ c) Viruses

_____ d) Spores

10. Is it safe to use a hospital disinfectant on stainless steel salon tools, and why or why not? _____

_____

_____

_____

_____

11. An item that is made of a material with no pores or openings and that cannot absorb liquids is considered _____.

12. When disinfecting your equipment, you should always choose a tuberculocidal disinfectant.

_____ True

_____ False

13. Before a manufacturer can sell a product for disinfecting tools, implements, or equipment, it must obtain a(n) _____ number that certifies that the disinfectant may be used in the manner prescribed by the manufacturer's label.

14. The EPA does not grade disinfectants.

_____ True

_____ False

15. A disinfectant approved for use on a countertop can also be assumed to be safe for use in a pedicure tub.

_____ True

_____ False

16. A state agency can issue penalties against both a salon owner and the cosmetologist's license.

_____ True

_____ False

17. What level of legislature writes laws to determine the scope of practice?

_____ a) Federal

_____ b) State

_____ c) Both a and b are correct.

_____ d) Neither a nor b is correct.

18. Laws are more specific than rules and regulations.

_____ True

_____ False

19. It is the responsibility of the cosmetologist to be aware of any changes or updates to the rules and regulations that apply to their work in the salon, and to comply with them.

_____ True

_____ False

PRINCIPLES OF INFECTION

20. If your actions result in an injury or infection, you could lose your license.

_____ True

_____ False

21. A _____ organism is one that is harmful to the human body.

22. An infectious disease may or may not be spread from one person to another person.

_____ True

_____ False

23. When you scrub something with soap and water or detergent and water to remove all visible dirt, debris, and many disease-causing germs, it is called:

_____ a) Cleaning

_____ b) Disinfecting

_____ c) Sterilizing

_____ d) Sanitizing

24. Disinfection destroys all organisms on environmental surfaces.

_____ True

_____ False

25. Disinfectants used in salons must be all BUT which of the following?

_____ a) Fungicidal

_____ b) Sporicidal

_____ c) Virucidal

_____ d) Bactericidal

26. When mixing and using a disinfectant, you must always follow the instructions on the label to ensure that it is used safely and effectively.

_____ True

_____ False

27. Contaminated salon tools and equipment can spread infections from client to client if the proper _____ steps are not taken after every service.

28. Where can bacteria exist?

_____

_____

_____

29. A surface is considered free of bacteria as long as it looks clean to the naked eye.

_____ True

_____ False

30. Differentiate between the two primary types of bacteria. _____

_____

_____

_____

_____

_____

31. Which type of bacteria causes pneumonia?

_____ a) Bacilli

_____ b) Staphylococci

_____ c) Diplococci

_____ d) Streptococci

32. Staphylococci:

_____ a) Are not pus-forming

_____ b) Grow in clusters like bunches of grapes

_____ c) Cause strep throat and blood poisoning

_____ d) Cause tetanus and typhoid fever

33. Bacteria and viruses produce toxins.

_____ True

_____ False

34. Which type of bacteria causes Lyme disease?

_____ a) Bacilli

_____ b) Staphylococci

_____ c) Spirilla

_____ d) Diplococci

35. All cocci use slender, hairlike extensions called flagella for locomotion.

_____ True

_____ False

36. Identify the three ways in which cocci are transmitted.

a) _____

b) _____

c) _____

37. Bacteria multiply best in cool, bright, dry places.

_____ True

_____ False

38. During the _____ or _____ stage, certain bacteria coat themselves with wax-like outer shells.

39. What are the five signs of inflammation?

a) _____

b) _____

c) _____

d) _____

e) _____

40. An abscess is an example of a _____.

41. Staphylococci are a relatively rare form of bacteria that can affect humans.

_____ True

_____ False

42. Staph bacteria can be picked up on doorknobs, countertops, and other surfaces.

_____ True

_____ False

43. How does MRSA commonly manifest and evolve (if left untreated)? _____

_____

_____

44. A(n) _____ is a reaction due to extreme sensitivity to certain foods, chemicals, or other normally harmless substances.

45. Contact with nonintact (broken) skin, blood, body fluid, or other potentially infectious materials as a result of the performance of employee duties is known as:

_____ a) Infectious disease

_____ b) Decontamination

_____ c) Exposure incident

_____ d) Inflammation

46. Lice and mites cause what type of disease?

_____ a) Pathogenic

_____ b) Parasitic

_____ c) Systemic

_____ d) Viral

47. A virus can replicate only by taking over the host cell's reproductive function.

_____ True

_____ False

48. Viral infections can be treated with antibiotics.

_____ True

_____ False

49. Which of the following is a sign of HPV infection?

_____ a) Small black dots on the bottom of the foot

_____ b) Redness and swelling around a healing wound

_____ c) Yellowing of the eyes

_____ d) Yellowing of the toenails

50. It is strongly recommended that cosmetologists be vaccinated for which strain of hepatitis?

_____ a) Hepatitis A

_____ b) Hepatitis B

_____ c) Hepatitis C

_____ d) Hepatitis D

51. Cosmetologists cannot cut live skin, but they are authorized to remove calluses.

_____ True

_____ False

52. In general, it is easy to contract hepatitis.

_____ True

_____ False

53. Explain how HIV spreads. _____

_____

_____

54. If you accidentally cut a client who is HIV-positive, the tool must be discarded and never used again.

_____ True

_____ False

55. Mildew is a common cause of human infections in the salon.

_____ True

_____ False

56. The most frequently encountered fungal infection resulting from hair services is tinea barbae, commonly known as _____.

57. It is recommended that you use _____ to quickly remove visible hair and debris from clippers.

58. Discuss how nail infections are spread. _____

_____

_____

59. Tinea pedis is a _____ fungus of the foot.

60. Head lice are a type of parasite responsible for contagious diseases and conditions.

_____ True

_____ False

61. Contagious diseases and conditions caused by parasites should only be treated by a doctor.

_____ True

_____ False

62. _____ immunity is partly inherited and partly developed through healthy living, while _____ immunity is immunity that the body develops after overcoming a disease, through inoculation, or through exposure to natural allergens.

PRINCIPLES OF PREVENTION

63. Describe the two methods of decontamination. _____

_____

_____

64. List three ways to clean tools or implements in Decontamination Method 1.

a) _____

_____

b) _____

c) _____

65. All tools and implements can be sterilized.

_____ True

_____ False

66. Using disinfectants as hand cleaners can cause skin irritation and _____, a reaction due to extreme sensitivity to certain foods, chemicals, or other normally harmless substances.

67. When mixing a disinfectant concentrate and water, you:

_____ a) Pour the water and disinfectant concentrate into a third container simultaneously

_____ b) Always add the water to the disinfectant concentrate

_____ c) Always add the disinfectant concentrate to the water

_____ d) Can combine the two substances in any order you choose

68. Identify and describe the accepted method for testing an autoclave. _____

_____

_____

_____

_____

69. Salons should keep an autoclave logbook for the state board to inspect. What three types of information about the autoclave should this logbook contain?

a) _____

b) _____

c) _____

70. All disinfectants have the same concentration.

_____ True

_____ False

71. _____, when applied to disinfectant claims, means the effectiveness with which a disinfecting solution kills organisms when used according to the label instructions.

72. List the characteristics of the ideal disinfectant.

a) _____

b) _____

c) _____

d) _____

e) _____

f) _____

g) _____

h) _____

i) _____

j) _____

73. If bleach is used to disinfect surfaces or equipment, it is critical to use soap or a detergent first to thoroughly clean the surface or equipment and remove all debris.

_____ True

_____ False

74. List the eight recommended tips for using disinfectants.

a) _____

b) _____

_____

c) _____

_____

d) _____

_____

e) _____

_____

_____

f) _____

_____

g) _____

h) _____

_____

_____

75. What are quats? _____

_____

76. Quat solutions usually disinfect surfaces and implements in?

_____ a) 5 minutes

_____ b) 10 minutes

_____ c) 15 minutes

_____ d) 20 minutes

77. Phenolic disinfectants:

_____ a) Are completely safe for the environment

_____ b) Are not tuberculocidal

_____ c) Have a very low pH

_____ d) Are a form of formaldehyde

78. Fumigants are a type of disinfectant commonly used in salons today.

_____ True

_____ False

79. What are the two main advantages of the disinfectant accelerated hydrogen peroxide (AHP)?

a) _____

b) _____

80. The technical term for household bleach is _____.

81. Explain how to mix a bleach solution. _____

_____

_____

_____

_____

_____

82. Explain why formalin tablets are no longer used in the salon. _____

_____

_____

_____

_____

_____

83. What are the nine things you should always do when using disinfectants?

a) _____

b) _____

c) _____

d) _____

e) _____

_____

f) _____

g) _____

_____

h) _____

_____

i) _____

_____

84. What are the two things you should never do when using disinfectants?

a) _____

b) _____

85. Multi use items must have hard, nonporous surfaces.

_____ True

_____ False

86. Single-use items cannot be properly cleaned so that all visible residue is removed.

_____ True

_____ False

87. What are three examples of multi use tools? _____

_____

_____

88. Define the term *porous*. _____

_____

89. Some porous items can be safely cleaned, disinfected, and used again.

_____ True

_____ False

90. If you are not sure if an item can be safely cleaned, disinfected, and used again, what should you do? _____

91. List seven examples of single-use items.

a) _____

b) _____

c) _____

d) _____

e) _____

f) _____

g) _____

92. Electric sterilizers and bead sterilizers can be used to effectively disinfect and sterilize implements.

_____ True

_____ False

UNIVERSAL PRECAUTIONS

93. The term _____ refers to guidelines published by OSHA that require employers and employees to assume that all human blood and body fluids are infectious for bloodborne pathogens.

94. Define the term *asymptomatic*. _____

_____

95. What are the three main precautions that protect salon employees in situations in which they could be exposed to bloodborne pathogens?

a) _____

b) _____

c) _____

_____

96. If a client suffers a cut or an abrasion that bleeds during a service, what should the salon professional do?

a) _____

b) _____

c) _____

_____

d) _____

e) _____

f) _____

_____

g) _____

_____

h) _____

_____

_____

_____

_____

i) _____

_____

_____

_____

j) _____

_____

PROFESSIONAL SALON IMAGE

97. List the 22 recommended guidelines for keeping a salon looking its best.

a) _____

b) _____

c) _____

d) _____

e) _____

f) _____

g) _____

_____

h) _____

i) _____

j) _____

_____

k) _____

l) _____

m) _____

n) _____

o) _____

_____

p) _____

q) _____

r) _____

s) _____

t) _____

u) _____

_____

_____

v) _____

98. The cosmetologist is professionally and legally responsible for following state and federal laws and rules.

_____ True

_____ False

DISINFECTION PROCEDURES

99. State regulations require that all tools and equipment be _____ and _____ before and after every service.

100. List the seven steps involved in disinfecting nonelectrical tools and equipment.

a) _____

b) _____

_____

c) _____

_____

d) _____

_____

e) _____

_____

f) _____

g) _____

_____

101. To prevent capes used for cutting, shampooing, and chemical services from touching a client's skin, use _____.

102. Explain how to clean and disinfect electrical equipment. _____

_____

_____

_____

_____

_____

_____

_____

103. Outline the procedure to follow after each client has used a whirlpool foot spa or air-jet basin.

a) _____

b) _____

_____

c) _____

d) _____

_____

_____

_____

e) _____

_____

104. At the end of every day, what should the cosmetologist do to disinfect units with footplates, impellers, impeller assemblies, and propellers?

a) _____

_____

_____

b) _____

c) _____

_____

_____

d) _____

_____

105. List the steps to take at the end of every day to disinfect nonwhirlpool foot basins or tubs.

a) _____

b) _____

_____

c) _____

_____

_____

d) _____

_____

106. Discuss the action and use of chelating soaps. _____

_____

_____

_____

_____

_____

107. Additives, powders, and tablets can eliminate the need to clean and disinfect.

_____ True

_____ False

108. If you cannot disinfect an item, you should _____ the item.

109. _____ is one of the most important actions you can take to prevent germs from spreading from one person to another.

110. Medical studies suggest that antimicrobial and antibacterial soaps are no more effective than regular soaps and detergents.

_____ True

_____ False

111. What is the procedure for proper hand washing?

a) _____

_____

_____

b) _____

_____

_____

_____

_____

c) _____

_____

d) _____

112. _____ are agents formulated for use on skin.

CHAPTER 6 General Anatomy and Physiology

See Milady Standard Cosmetology Theory Workbook.

CHAPTER 7 Skin Structure, Growth, and Nutrition

See Milady Standard Cosmetology Theory Workbook.

CHAPTER 8 Skin Disorders and Diseases

See Milady Standard Cosmetology Theory Workbook.

CHAPTER 9 Nail Structure and Growth

See Milady Standard Cosmetology Theory Workbook.

CHAPTER 10 Nail Disorders and Diseases

See Milady Standard Cosmetology Theory Workbook.

CHAPTER 11 Properties of the Hair and Scalp

See Milady Standard Cosmetology Theory Workbook.

CHAPTER 12 Basics of Chemistry

See Milady Standard Cosmetology Theory Workbook.

CHAPTER 13 Basics of Electricity

See Milady Standard Cosmetology Theory Workbook.

CHAPTER 14 Principles of Hair Design

See Milady Standard Cosmetology Theory Workbook.

15 Scalp Care, Shampooing, and Conditioning

Date: _____

Rating: _____

Text Pages: 306–341

POINT TO PONDER:

"The highest reward for your work is not what you get for it, but what you become by it."—**John C. Maxwell**

1. The shampoo is one of the most important experiences a stylist provides.

   _____ True

   _____ False

2. What are the three processes of the shampoo?

   a) _____

   b) _____

   c) _____

WHY STUDY SCALP CARE, SHAMPOOING, AND CONDITIONING?

3. In your own words, explain why cosmetologists should study and thoroughly understand scalp care, shampooing, and conditioning. _____

_____

_____

_____

_____

_____

_____

_____

SCALP CARE AND MASSAGE

4. The two basic requirements for a healthy scalp are _____ and _____ .

5. Scalp manipulations should be given with a _____ motion, which will _____ the scalp and help _____ the client.

6. The cosmetologist can massage or manipulate a client's scalp when abrasions are present.

_____ True

_____ False

7. Scalp treatments and massage may be performed before or during a shampoo.

_____ True

_____ False

8. The difference between a relaxation massage and a treatment massage are the products used.

_____ True

_____ False

9. During the scalp-massage consultation, the cosmetologist should acknowledge and discuss any procedure or condition that may be _____ because it may produce undesirable side effects.

10. Scalp massage is contraindicated for clients with which of the following?

_____ a. Circulatory condition

_____ b. Severe hypertension

_____ c. High blood pressure

_____ d. Diabetes

11. Cosmetologists who talk during scalp massage enhance the procedure's relaxation therapy.

_____ True

_____ False

12. The pre-service procedure is an organized, step-by-step plan for what three tasks?

a. _____

b. _____

c. _____

13. List the three major tasks of the post-service procedure.

a. _____

b. _____

c. _____

14. Explain how to commence the scalp massage procedure. _____

_____

_____

15. What does the following illustration depict? _____

_____

16. Discuss the purpose of a general scalp treatment and when it should be recommended. _____

_____

_____

17. Outline the procedure for a normal hair and scalp treatment.

a. _____

_____

b. _____

c. _____

d. _____

e. _____

_____

f. _____

g. _____

h. _____

i. _____

j. _____

k. _____

l. _____

_____

18. Outline the special requirements and implements of a dry hair and scalp treatment. _____

_____

_____

_____

_____

_____

19. During a dry hair and scalp treatment, apply the scalp steamer for _____ to _____ minutes, or wrap the head in warm steam towels for _____ to _____ minutes.

20. Excessive oiliness is caused by _____.

21. List the implements and materials for an oily hair and scalp treatment.

a. _____

b. _____

c. _____

d. _____

e. _____

f. _____

g. _____

h. _____

i. _____

j. _____

22. _____ is the result of a fungus called malassezia.

23. Detail the steps in an antidandruff treatment.

a. _____

_____

b. _____

c. _____

d. _____

e. _____

f. _____

g. _____

h. _____

_____

i. _____

j. _____

HAIR BRUSHING

24. What are the benefits of correct hair brushing? _____

_____

_____

_____

25. When should a stylist avoid brushing hair?

a. _____

b. _____

26. Brushing, massaging, or shampooing the scalp before a service is not recommended for:

a. _____

b. _____

c. _____

d. _____

27. The most highly recommended hairbrushes are made from _____ bristles.

28. Hairbrushes with _____ bristles are shiny and smooth and are more suitable for hairstyling.

29. Name the steps in the hair brushing procedure.

a. _____

_____

b. _____

c. _____

d. _____

e. _____

f. _____

g. _____

h. _____

i. _____

_____

j. _____

_____

k. _____

l. _____

m. _____

UNDERSTANDING SHAMPOO

30. Name the conditions for which the stylist should check when performing a shampoo.

a. _____

b. _____

c. _____

d. _____

e. _____

f. _____

g. _____

h. _____

i. _____

31. Hair should only be shampooed as often as necessary.

_____ True

_____ False

32. Excessive shampooing strips the hair of its protective oil, called _____, which, in small amounts, seals and protects the hair's cuticle.

33. As a general rule, oily hair must be shampooed less often than normal or dry hair.

_____ True

_____ False

34. Give the steps in the basic shampooing and conditioning procedure.

a. _____

_____

b. _____

_____

c. _____

_____

d. _____

e. _____

f. _____

_____

_____

g. _____

_____

_____

_____

h. _____

35. Why is it important to maintain good posture while performing a shampoo?

_____

_____

_____

36. What is the most important rule regarding posture while shampooing, and why?

_____

_____

37. What type of shampoo bowl allows for healthier body alignment and helps reduce back and shoulder strain? _____

_____

38. List the typical types of hair.

a. _____

b. _____

c. _____

d. _____

39. Chemically treated hair may require products that are _____ _____than those for virgin hair.

40. The amount of _____ in a solution determines whether that solution is alkaline or acid.

41. A shampoo that is acidic will have a pH ranging from ____ to _____.

42. The more alkaline a shampoo, the stronger and harsher it is.

_____ True

_____ False

43. _____ is the most abundant and important element on Earth.

44. Why is water classified as a universal solvent? _____

_____

_____

45. Boiling water at a temperature of _____ degrees Fahrenheit will destroy most microbes.

46. _____ water is rainwater or chemically treated water that contains only small amounts of minerals, while _____ water contains minerals that reduce the ability of soap or shampoo to lather.

47. The main ingredient in most shampoos is _____ water, which has had impurities like calcium and other metal ions removed.

48. _____, also known as detergents, are cleansing or surface active agents.

49. The end of a molecule that attracts water is called _____, while the oil-attracting end is called _____.

50. Shampoo products are the most widely purchased of all hair care products.

_____ True

_____ False

51. Many shampoos are balanced by adding _____, _____, or _____ acid.

52. _____ shampoos are designed to make hair manageable and smooth and shiny.

53. Give two examples of conditioning agents that boost shampoos.

a. _____

b. _____

54. Clarifying shampoos contain an active _____ agent that binds to metals and removes them from hair, as well as a(n) _____ agent that enriches hair, helps retain moisture, and makes hair more manageable.

55. Explain when clarifying shampoos should be used. _____

_____

_____

56. For oily hair and scalp, _____ shampoos wash away excess oiliness while preventing the hair from drying out.

57. A(n) _____ or _____ shampoo cleanses hair without soap and water.

58. A dry shampoo removes volume from hair.

_____ True

_____ False

59. Discuss the ways in which color-enhancing shampoos are used.

_____

_____

60. Describe shampooing for wheelchair-bound clients. _____

_____

_____

_____

_____

61. What implements and materials are required for a basic shampoo?

a) _____

b) _____

c) _____

d) _____

e) _____

f) _____

g) _____

62. List the steps for a shampoo procedure.

a) _____

b) _____

c) _____

d) _____

e) _____

f) _____

g) _____

_____

_____

h) _____

_____

i) _____

_____

j) _____

_____

k) _____

_____

l) _____

_____

_____

m) _____

_____

n) _____

_____

o) _____

_____

p) _____

_____

q) _____

r) _____

_____

s) _____

_____

t) _____

u) _____

v) _____

_____

w) _____

x) _____

y) _____

_____

_____

z) _____

aa) _____

_____

_____

bb) _____

_____

_____

cc) _____

dd) _____

ee) _____

_____

UNDERSTANDING CONDITIONER

63. Why are conditioners used? _____

_____

_____

64. Name the three basic types of conditioner.

a. _____

b. _____

c. _____

65. Most conditioners contain silicone, along with moisture-binding _____, substances that absorb moisture or promote the retention of moisture.

66. The cortex makes up _____ percent of the hair strand.

67. Identify some conditioning agents and their uses.

a. _____

_____

_____

b. _____

c. _____

d. _____

_____

68. _____, also known as hair masks or conditioning packs, are chemical mixtures of concentrated protein and intensive moisturizer.

DRAPING

69. Client draping contributes to client safety as well as comfort.

_____ True

_____ False

70. Name the two types of drapings used in salons.

a. _____

b. _____

71. Explain when and how a shampoo draping is used. _____

_____

_____

_____

_____

_____

_____

72. When is a chemical draping used? _____

_____

_____

_____

73. List the steps to draping for a chemical service.

a. _____

_____

b. _____

_____

c. _____

_____

d. _____

e. _____

_____

_____

16 Haircutting

Date: _____

Rating: _____

Text Pages: 342–417

POINT TO PONDER:

"It is right to be content with what you have, but not with what you are."—**Unknown**

WHY STUDY HAIRCUTTING?

1. In your own words, explain why cosmetologists should study and thoroughly understand haircutting. _____

_____

_____

_____

_____

_____

_____

_____

BASIC PRINCIPLES OF HAIRCUTTING

2. Good haircuts begin with an understanding of the _____, referred to as _____.

3. To help achieve the look that you and your client are seeking, be aware of where the head form _____.

4. _____ on the head mark where the surface of the head changes.

5. List common reference points.

   a) _____

   b) _____

   c) _____

   d) _____

6. An understanding of head shape and reference points will help the cosmetologist:

a) _____

b) _____

c) _____

_____

7. Match each of the following reference points with its description.

_____ 1. Parietal ridge   a) Highest point on the top of the head

_____ 2. Occipital bone   b) Widest area of the head, starting at the temples and ending at the bottom of the crown

_____ 3. Apex   c) Front and back corner of the head

_____ 4. Four corners   d) Bone that protrudes at the base of the skull

8. How can you find the parietal ridge?_____

_____

9. Describe how to find the occipital bone. _____

_____

10. Explain how to find the apex. _____

_____

11. Outline two ways to find the four corners._____

_____

_____

_____

12. Name the areas of the head.

a) _____

b) _____

c) _____

d) _____

e) _____

f) _____

g) _____

13. Why is the top of the head important to identify? _____

_____

_____

_____

14. Give the procedure for determining the front of the head. _____

_____

_____

_____

15. Where are the sides of the head? _____

_____

16. What is the crown, and why is it important to identify? _____

_____

_____

_____

17. What is the nape, and how can it be identified? _____

_____

_____

_____

18. What does the back of the head consist of? Explain how to locate it. _____

_____

_____

19. Define the bang or fringe area. _____

_____

20. A(n) _____ is a thin, continuous mark used as a guide.

21. A(n) _____ is the space between two lines or surfaces that intersect at a
given point.

22. The two basic lines used in haircutting are:

a) _____

b) _____

23. Label the three types of straight lines in the accompanying figure:

a) _____

b) _____

c) _____

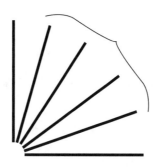

24. Horizontal lines are _____ to the horizon or the floor. They _____ weight and are used to create _____ and _____ haircuts.

25. Vertical lines are _____ to the floor. They _____ weight, are used to create _____ or _____ haircuts, and are used with _____ _____.

26. Diagonal lines, which have a(n) _____ direction, are used to create _____ and to blend _____.

27. _____ techniques use diagonal lines to create angles by cutting the ends of the hair with a slight increase or decrease in length.

28. Angles are important elements in haircutting because they _____ _____.

29. For control during haircutting, the hair is parted into uniform working areas called _____. Each section may be divided into smaller partings called _____.

30. The line dividing the hair at the scalp, separating one section of hair from another, is called a(n) _____ or _____.

31. _____ is the angle or degree at which a subsection of hair is held or elevated from the head when cutting.

32. In a blunt cut or one-length haircut, what degree of elevation is employed?

_____ a) 90

_____ b) 45

_____ c) 30

_____ d) 0

33. What are the two most commonly used elevations in haircutting?

a) _____

b) _____

34. The more you elevate the hair, the more _____.

35. When you elevate hair below 90 degrees, you _____.

36. When you elevate hair above 90 degrees, you _____.

37. _____ is when hair contracts or lifts through the action of moisture loss/ drying.

38. The _____ is the angle at which the fingers are held when cutting the line that creates the end shape.

39. Give other names for the term *cutting* line.

a) _____

b) _____

c) _____

d) _____

40. Cutting lines can be described as:

a) _____

b) _____

c) _____

d) _____

41. Define the term *guideline*. _____

_____

42. The _____ of a cut is the outer line, while the _____ is the inner or internal line of the cut.

43. What are the two types of guidelines in haircutting?

a) _____

b) _____

44. A guideline that does not move during haircutting is considered _____.

45. A guideline that moves as a haircut progresses is classified as _____.

46. What is overdirection, and why is it used? _____

_____

_____

_____

_____

_____

CLIENT CONSULTATION

47. A(n) _____ is a conversation between the cosmetologist and client during which the cosmetologist determines what the client is looking for, offers suggestions and professional advice, and reaches a joint decision with the client about the most suitable haircut.

48. Explain how to analyze face shape. _____

_____

_____

_____

49. What does analyzing face shape accomplish? _____

_____

_____

50. When analyzing face shape, an important point to consider is the client's _____, or how the client looks from the side.

51. A haircut should flatter a client by emphasizing good features, like a(n) _____, and de-emphasizing less-flattering features, like a(n) _____.

52. As it dries, hair will shrink _____ inch to _____ inch.

_____ a) ⅛, ¼

_____ b) ¼ , ½

_____ c) ½, ¾

_____ d) ¾, 1

53. What four characteristics determine the behavior of hair?

a) _____

b) _____

c) _____

d) _____

54. The _____ is the hair that grows at the outermost perimeter along the face, around the ears, and on the neck.

55. The growth pattern is the direction in which the hair grows from the scalp, also called the _____ or the _____.

56. You may need to use _____ tension when cutting cowlicks, whorls, and other growth patterns.

_____ a) More

_____ b) Less

57. The number of individual hair strands on 1 square inch (2.5 square cm) of scalp is known as _____.

58. _____, usually classified as coarse, medium, or fine, is based on the thickness or diameter of each strand.

59. Why are density and texture important? _____

_____

_____

60. The _____, or amount of movement in a hair strand, can be straight, wavy, curly, extremely curly, or anything in between.

HAIRCUTTING TOOLS

61. Match each of the following tools with its most common haircutting use.

_____ Haircutting shears   a) Achieve softer effect on hair ends

_____ Texturizing shears   b) Remove excess or unwanted neckline hair

_____ Razors   c) Cut close tapers on the nape and sides

_____ Clippers   d) Detangle hair

_____ Trimmers   e) Cut blunt or straight lines

_____ Sectioning clips   f) Section and subsection hair

_____ Wide-tooth comb   g) Support most procedures

_____ Tail comb   h) Keep portions of hair separate

_____ Barber comb   i) Create short haircuts and tapers

_____ Styling or cutting comb   j) Remove bulk

62. Which three countries are primarily responsible for manufacturing the steel used to make professional shears?

a) _____

b) _____

c) _____

63. Generally, a shear with a Rockwell hardness of at least _____ or _____ is ideal.

64. As the hardness of steel increases, its ability to retain a sharp edge:

_____ a) Increases

_____ b) Decreases

_____ c) Remains the same

65. A(n) _____ shear is made by pouring molten steel into a mold, whereas a(n) _____ shear is made by hammering or pressing metal to a finished shape.

66. Compare forged shears with cast ones. _____

_____

_____

_____

_____

67. Match each of the following shear parts with its function.

_____ Cutting edge   a) Afford shear control

_____ Pivot and adjustment area   b) Achieve cutting

_____ Adjustment knob   c) Make shears cut

_____ Finger tang   d) Control blade tension

68. List all the tasks that should be on the shears' maintenance schedule.

a) _____

b) _____

c) _____

d) _____

e) _____

69. A left-hand cutter can use a right-handed shear by simply turning the shear over.

_____ a) True

_____ b) False

70. Name the things a cosmetologist should do when considering a shears purchase.

a) _____

b) _____

c) _____

d) _____

e) _____

f) _____

g) _____

h) _____

i) _____

j) _____

71. When purchasing shears, a full _____ edge will give the smoothest cut, while a(n) _____ edge is dull and can be noisy.

72. Which of the following types of shears adds increased blending?

_____ a) Chunking

_____ b) Texturizing

_____ c) Thinning

_____ d) Blending

73. Ergonomically correct and custom-fitted shears can help the cosmetologist dramatically by:

a) _____

b) _____

c) _____

74. List the four components of correctly fitting a shear.

a) _____

b) _____

c) _____

d) _____

75. It is important to hold tools properly because doing so:

a) _____

b) _____

76. Describe the proper way to hold shears.

a) _____

_____

b) _____

c) _____

_____

77. Why is it important to always hold the comb while cutting? _____

_____

78. Differentiate between the roles of the dominant hand and the holding hand during haircutting. _____

_____

_____

_____

79. Explain what it means to "palm the shears." _____

_____

_____

_____

80. Define the phrase "transferring the comb." _____

_____

_____

_____

81. A(n) _____, or feather blade, is a versatile tool that can be used for an entire haircut.

82. Describe the two methods of holding a razor.

Method A

a) _____

_____

Method B

a) _____

b) _____

83. In a comb, _____ teeth are used for combing and parting hair, while _____ teeth comb a section before cutting.

84. In haircutting, _____ is the amount of pressure applied when combing and holding a subsection.

85. Why is consistent tension important in haircutting? _____

_____

POSTURE AND BODY POSITION

86. What steps can you take to ensure you are using good posture and body positioning when cutting hair?

a) _____

b) _____

c) _____

87. List the hand positions for different cutting angles and when they are used.

a) _____

_____

b) _____

_____

c) _____

SAFETY IN HAIRCUTTING

88. What precautions should you take when handling sharp tools and instruments?

a) _____

b) _____

_____

c) _____

d) _____

_____

_____

e) _____

f) _____

BASIC HAIRCUTS

89. Name the four basic haircuts.

a) _____

b) _____

c) _____

d) _____

90. In a(n) _____ cut, also known as a one-length haircut, all the hair comes to one hanging level, forming a weight line.

91. What is a weight line? _____

_____

92. The cutting line in a blunt cut can be:

_____ a) Horizontal

_____ b) Diagonal

_____ c) Rounded

_____ d) All of these answers are correct.

93. The most common elevation in a graduated haircut is _____ degrees.

_____ a) 180

_____ b) 90

_____ c) 45

_____ d) 0

94. A(n) _____ haircut is a graduated effect achieved by cutting the hair with elevation or overdirection.

95. A layered haircut is cut at higher elevations, usually _____ degrees and above.

_____ a) 180

_____ b) 90

_____ c) 45

_____ d) 0

96. A long-layered haircut is cut at a _____-degree angle.

_____ a) 180

_____ b) 90

_____ c) 45

_____ d) 0

97. Describe the shape of a long-layered haircut. _____

_____

98. List general haircutting tips.

a) _____

b) _____

c) _____

d) _____

e) _____

f) _____

g) _____

h) _____

i) _____

j) _____

k) _____

99. _____ is parting the haircut in the opposite way that you cut it to check for precision of line and shape.

100. Give some alternate names for the blunt cut. _____

_____

101. For a blunt cut, the client's head should be in what position? _____

_____

102. What happens when a client's head is improperly positioned for a blunt cut?

a) _____

b) _____

103. Outline the pre-service procedure for cleaning and disinfecting.

a) _____

b) _____

c) _____

d) _____

_____

e) _____

_____

f) _____

g) _____

h) _____

104. Give the pre-service procedural steps for basic station setup.

a) _____

b) _____

_____

c) _____

_____

105. Explain how a stylist would prepare for a service.

a) _____

_____

b) _____

c) _____

d) _____

e) _____

f) _____

106. Outline the procedure for greeting a client.

a) _____

_____

b) _____

c) _____

107. Name the three main parts of the post-service procedure.

a) _____

b) _____

c) _____

108. Identify the implements and materials needed for the blunt cut with fringe.

a) _____

b) _____

c) _____

d) _____

e) _____

f) _____

g) _____

h) _____

i) _____

j) _____

109. How should the hair be parted when cutting a blunt cut with fringe?

_____

_____

110. Where do you begin a blunt haircut with fringe? _____

_____

_____

111. How should you create your guideline for a right-handed blunt cut with fringe?

_____

_____

_____

_____

_____

_____

_____

112. When cutting the crown area in a blunt cut with fringe, what should you pay close attention to? _____

_____

_____

113. When working left-handed, how should you match the sides of the blunt haircut with fringe to the back? _____

_____

_____

114. Discuss some danger areas with blunt cuts. _____

_____

_____

_____

_____

115. In a classic A-line bob, a(n) _____ cutting line is used.

116. In a classic pageboy, the perimeter is _____.

117. List tips for blunt haircuts.

a) _____

b) _____

c) _____

d) _____

e) _____

f) _____

118. For the _____ haircut, you work with a vertical cutting line and a 45-degree elevation, as well as a 90-degree elevation.

119. For the graduated haircut, the hair is parted into _____ sections.

120. Describe the action taking place in the following illustrations of a right-handed graduated haircut:

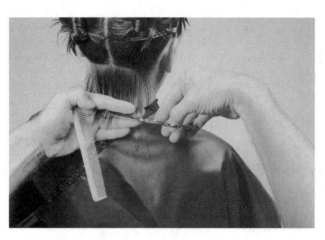

_____

_____

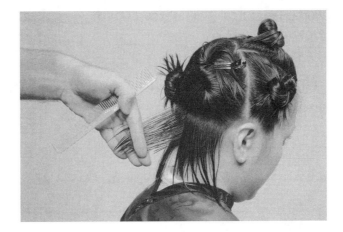

121. As you continue throughout the left and right sections of a graduated haircut, the hair becomes gradually _____ as it reaches the apex.

122. Describe the action taking place in the following illustrations of a left-handed graduated haircut:

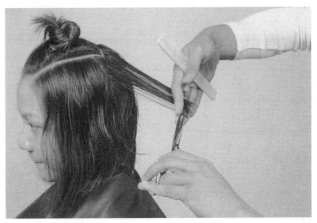

_____

_____

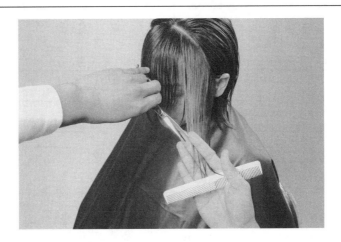

_____

123. In a uniform-layered haircut, all hair is elevated to _____ degrees and cut at the same length, using a(n) _____ guideline that is inside the haircut rather than on the perimeter.

124. How can you maintain control and consistency while working through a uniform-layered haircut? _____

_____

_____

_____

125. Describe the concept of increased layering. _____

_____

_____

_____

126. List the steps involved in completing a long-layered haircut left-handed.

a) _____

b) _____

_____

c) _____

d) _____

e) _____

_____

f) _____

g) _____

_____

    a. _____

    b. _____

_____

h) _____

i) _____

j) _____

_____

k) _____

OTHER CUTTING TECHNIQUES

127. What is important to remember when cutting curly hair? _____

_____

_____

128. Curly hair _____ much more than straight hair after drying. For every ¼ inch (0.6 cm) you cut when the hair is wet, it will shrink up to _____ inch (cm) when dry.

129. Why should you use minimal tension when cutting curly hair? _____

_____

_____

130. What is the effect of using a razor on curly hair? _____

_____

131. The _____ or _____ area is the hair that lies between the two front corners, or approximately between the outer corners of the eyes.

132. What is meant by distribution? _____

_____

133. What factor determines whether hair in the bang area must blend with the rest of the haircut? _____

134. A razor cut gives a _____ appearance than a shear cut.

135. Differentiate between a shear cut and a razor cut. _____

_____

_____

136. A razor guide is _____ your fingers, whereas the guide with shears is usually _____ your fingers.

137. Why should you always use a new, sharp blade when razor cutting? _____

_____

138. List tips for cutting with a razor.

a) _____

b) _____

c) _____

d) _____

e) _____

139. Slide cutting is useful for:

a) _____

b) _____

c) _____

140. How is slide cutting accomplished? _____

_____

141. _____ is a technique in which you hold the hair in place with a comb while using the tips of shears to remove length.

142. The scissor-over-comb technique is generally used to:

a) _____

b) _____

143. List the basic steps of the shears-over-comb technique.

a) _____

_____

b) _____

_____

c) _____

_____

_____

d) _____

_____

144. _____ is the process of removing excess bulk without shortening length.

145. Texturizing techniques can be used to:

a) _____

b) _____

c) _____

d) _____

146. What tools are used for texturizing? _____

_____

147. Match each of the following texturizing techniques with the phrase that best describes it.

_____ 1. Point cutting   a) Performed on hair ends using shear tips

_____ 2. Notching   b) Thins hair to graduated lengths with shears

_____ 3. Free-hand notching   c) Removes bulk and adds movement through lengths of hair

_____ 4. Slithering   d) Aggressive means of creating a chunky effect

_____ 5. Slicing   s) Creates visual separation in hair

_____ 6. Carving   f) Used on the interior of a section to release curl and remove density

148. How do thinning shears remove weight from a haircut? _____

_____

_____

149. What is the razor rotation technique used for? _____

_____

CLIPPERS AND TRIMMERS

150. What are clippers? _____

_____

151. Clippers are good for cutting shorter haircuts and can be used to create _____, which sit very close to the hairline and gradually get longer as you move up the head.

152. Identify the ways in which clippers can be used.

a) _____

b) _____

_____

c) _____

153. List all the tools to have on hand when clipper cutting.

a) _____

b) _____

c) _____

d) _____

e) _____

154. The _____ technique allows you to cut very close to the scalp and create a flat-top or square shape.

155. Clippers are more accurate when used on _____ hair.

156. Using length guard attachments is a quick and easy way to create _____ haircuts.

157. Always work against the natural growth pattern when cutting with clippers.

_____ True

_____ False

158. When using the clipper-over-comb technique, the angle at which you hold the comb determines the _____.

159. How should you part the hair for a clipper cut? _____

_____

_____

160. Where and how should you begin the clipper cut? _____

_____

_____

_____

161. How do you blend the sections with clippers? _____

_____

_____

162. To cut the hair very close from the sideburn to the parietal ridge, you should use a _____ attachment.

163. How should you determine the guideline for the length in the crown area?

_____

_____

164. Clippers and trimmers can be used to trim beards and mustaches.

_____ True

_____ False

CHAPTER 17 Hairstyling

Date: _____

Rating: _____

Text Pages: 418–505

POINT TO PONDER:

"Time is usually wasted in the same way every day."—**Paul Meyer**

WHY STUDY HAIRSTYLING?

1. In your own words, explain why cosmetologists should study and thoroughly understand hairstyling.

_____

_____

_____

_____

_____

_____

_____

CLIENT CONSULTATION

2. What is the best way for clients to convey their expectations in terms of hairstyle preference? _____

_____

3. What factors will help determine the best hairstyle? _____

_____

WET HAIRSTYLING BASICS

4. List commonly used wet hairstyling tools.

a) _____

b) _____

c) _____

d) _____

e) _____

f) _____

FINGER WAVING

5. Finger waving is the process of _____
_____ through the use of the fingers, combs, and waving lotion.

6. Why should cosmetologists learn finger waving of the 1920s and 1930s?

_____

_____

_____

_____

7. _____ is a type of hair gel that makes the hair pliable enough to
keep it in place during the finger-waving procedure.

8. Waving lotion is traditionally made from _____, taken from trees found
in _____ and _____.

9. How will you know if you have used too much waving lotion on the hair?

_____

10. How do vertical finger waves differ from horizontal finger waves?

_____

_____

PIN CURLS

11. _____ curls serve as the basis for patterns, lines, waves, and rolls that are
used in a wide range of hairstyles.

12. Pin curls can be used only on hair that has been permanently waved.

_____ True

_____ False

13. Pin curls work best when the hair is layered and smoothly wound.

_____ True

_____ False

14. Identify the three principal parts of pin curls.

a) _____

b) _____

c) _____

15. The _____ is the stationary (nonmoving) foundation of the curl, which is the area closest to the scalp.

16. The _____ is the section of the pin curl between the base and first arc (turn) of the circle that gives the circle its direction and movement.

17. The size of the _____, the hair that is wrapped around the roller, determines the width of the wave and its strength.

18. The _____ is the hair between the scalp and the first turn of the roller.

_____ a) Base

_____ b) Stem

_____ c) Circle

19. Curl mobility is classified as which of the following?

_____ a) No-stem

_____ b) Half-stem

_____ c) Full-stem

_____ d) All of these answers are correct.

20. The _____ curl is placed directly on the base of the curl; produces a tight, firm, long-lasting curl; and allows minimum mobility.

21. The _____ curl permits medium movement, is placed half off the base, and gives good control to the hair.

22. The _____ curl allows for the greatest mobility because it is placed completely off the base and gives as much freedom as the length of the stem will permit.

23. The base of a full-stem curl may be what shape? _____

_____

_____

24. A(n) _____ is a section of hair that is molded in a circular movement in preparation for the formation of curls.

25. Shapings are either _____ or _____.

26. _____ curls produce even, smooth waves and uniform curls.

27. _____ curls produce waves that get smaller toward the end.

28. What is a clockwise curl? _____

_____

29. What is a counterclockwise curl? _____

_____

30. What base shapes are used in pin curls?

a) _____

b) _____

c) _____

d) _____

31. To avoid splits in a finished hairstyle, use care when selecting and forming the

_____.

32. Where are rectangular base pin curls recommended? _____

_____

_____

33. Where are triangular base pin curls recommended? _____

_____

_____

34. Where are arc base pin curls used? _____

_____

35. When are square base pin curls used? _____

_____

36. To avoid splits when combing out a pin curl set, you should _____
the sectioning.

37. _____ is the technique that involves forcing the hair between the
thumb and the back of the comb to create tension.

_____ a) Threading

_____ b) Ribboning

_____ c) Slicing

_____ d) Sculpting

38. Pin curls sliced from a shaping and formed without lifting the hair from the head are called _____ curls, also known as _____ curls.

39. How are pin curls used to create ridge curls? _____

_____

40. What are skip waves? _____

_____

41. _____ curls have large center openings and are fastened to the head in a standing position on a rectangular base.

42. What effect do barrel curls give? _____

_____

43. What are cascade curls used for? _____

_____

44. How are cascade curls fastened? _____

_____

ROLLER CURLS

45. What advantages do rollers have over pin curls?

a) _____

b) _____

_____

c) _____

46. Identify the three parts of the roller curl.

a) _____

b) _____

c) _____

47. What is the function of the base in a roller curl? _____

_____

48. What is the appropriate size of a roller-curl base? _____

_____

49. In a roller curl, the _____ is the hair between the scalp and the first turn of the roller.

50. What is the function of the stem in a roller curl? _____

_____

51. In a roller curl, the _____ or circle is the hair that is wrapped around the roller.

52. Why is the size of a roller-curl circle important? _____

_____

53. Match the following type of curl with the number of times it is wound around the roller.

_____ One complete turn   a) Curls

_____ One and a half turns   b) C-shaped curl

_____ Two and a half turns   c) Wave

54. The amount of _____ that is achieved depends on the size of the roller and how it sits on its base.

55. An on-base curl will give _____ volume.

56. A half-base curl will give _____ volume.

57. A(n) _____ curl will give very little volume.

58. For versatility in styling, a(n) _____ directional wrap gives options to style in all directions while still maintaining volume.

59. _____ is the point where curls of opposite directions meet, forming a recessed area.

60. Hot rollers are to be used only on dry hair.

_____ True

_____ False

61. What type of client is best suited for a Velcro set? _____

_____

_____

62. Why do the state boards of some states and provinces disallow Velcro rollers?

_____

_____

63. How long do Velcro rollers stay in the hair? _____

_____

_____

COMB-OUT TECHNIQUES

64. What are the benefits of a well-structured system of combing out hairstyles?

_____

_____

65. What is the best way to lift and increase volume, as well as remove the indentations caused by roller setting? _____

_____

_____

66. List the alternative names for backcombing.

a) _____

b) _____

c) _____

d) _____

e) _____

67. What action is involved in backcombing? _____

_____

_____

68. _____ or ruffing is used to build a soft cushion or to mesh two or more curl patterns for a uniform and smooth comb out.

69. What are the main uses of backcombing and backbrushing? _____

_____

_____

70. List the steps of the procedure for backcombing.

a) _____

b) _____

c) _____

d) _____

e) _____

f) _____

71. Give the procedure for backbrushing.

a) _____

b) _____

c) _____

d) _____

e) _____

f) _____

72. When is a finishing spray applied during backbrushing? _____

_____

_____

HAIR WRAPPING

73. What is the goal of hair wrapping? _____

_____

74. When height is desired with hair wrapping, place large rollers _____

_____.

75. Wrapping can be done on wet hair only.

_____ True

_____ False

76. When wrapping very curly hair, the first step is to _____.

BLOWDRY STYLING

77. Blowdry styling is the technique of _____ and _____ damp hair in one operation.

78. A(n) _____ is an electrical appliance designed for drying and styling hair.

79. The blowdryer's nozzle attachment, or _____, is a directional feature that creates a concentrated stream of air.

80. The _____ of a blowdryer is an attachment that causes the air to flow more softly and helps to accentuate or keep textural definition.

81. What can happen when a blowdryer is unclean? _____

_____

82. Combs and picks are designed to _____ and _____ the hair.

83. Combs with teeth that are closely spaced _____ definition from the curl, thus creating a smooth surface.

84. Combs with wide spaces between teeth _____ larger sections of hair for a more textured surface.

85. Combs with picks at one end serve to _____.

86. Describe a classic styling brush: _____

_____

87. What are classic styling brushes best used for? _____

_____

88. Describe a paddle brush and what it is used for: _____

_____

89. _____ brushes are generally oval with a mixture of boar and nylon bristles.

90. In a grooming brush, _____ bristles help distribute the scalp oils over the hair shaft, giving it shine, while _____ bristles stimulate the circulation of blood to the scalp.

91. What are grooming brushes particularly useful for? _____

_____

_____

92. _____ brushes, with their ventilated design, are used to speed the blowdrying process and are ideal for blowdrying fine hair and adding lift at the scalp.

93. How are round brushes used? _____

_____

_____

94. Why do some round brushes have metal cylinder bases? _____

_____

_____

_____

95. A(n) _____ brush is a nylon styling brush that has a tail for sectioning, along with a narrow row of bristles.

96. How are teasing brushes used? _____

_____

_____

97. _____ clips are usually metal or plastic and have long prongs to hold wet or dry sections of hair in place.

98. Styling lotions can be thought of as _____ tools.

99. What options must stylists consider before applying styling products?

a) _____

b) _____

c) _____

d) _____

100. Foam builds _____ body and volume into hair.

101. How is mousse used? _____

_____

_____

102. Foam is good for which type of hair? _____

_____

103. What is the purpose of gel? _____

_____

_____

104. How do liquid gels relate to firm-hold gels? _____

_____

_____

105. Explain the effect of straightening gels. _____

_____

_____

106. When sprayed into the base of fine, wet hair that is then blown dry, _____ add volume, especially at the base.

107. _____, also known as wax, adds considerable weight to hair by causing strands to join.

108. Nonoily silicone products are excellent for all hair types.

_____ True

_____ False

109. Hair spray, also known as _____ spray, is applied in the form of a mist to hold a style in position.

110. Graduated haircuts have interiors with layers that are:

_____ a) Long

_____ b) Short

_____ c) Long and short

_____ d) None of these answers are correct.

THERMAL HAIRSTYLING

111. Thermal waving and curling is also called _____ waving.

112. What are thermal waving and curling? _____

_____

_____

113. Which stylists favor nonelectrical thermal irons, and why? _____

_____

_____

114. Name the four basic parts of a thermal iron.

a) _____

b) _____

c) _____

d) _____

115. Flat irons with straight edges are used to create _____ styles, even on very curly hair.

116. What is the best way to test an iron's temperature? _____

_____

_____

117. Describe how to remove dirt, oils, or product residue from a thermal iron:

_____

_____

_____

_____

118. The comb used with a thermal iron should be about _____ inches (cm) long.

_____ 3 (7.5 cm)

_____ 5 (12.5 cm)

_____ 7 (17.5 cm)

_____ 9 (22.5 cm)

119. Describe how to manipulate a thermal iron:

a) _____

b) _____

_____

c) _____

_____

_____

120. What factor determines the correct temperature for thermal styling?

_____

_____

121. As a rule, coarse and gray hair can withstand _____ heat than fine hair.

122. Why is thermal curling used on straight hair? _____

_____

_____

123. Thermal curling cannot be used on human hair wigs and hairpieces.

_____ True

_____ False

124. What is the key to becoming good at using curling irons? _____

_____

125. Developing a smooth, _____ movement is important in thermal curling.

126. When practicing with thermal irons, guiding the hair strand into the center of the curl as you rotate the irons helps ensure that _____

_____.

127. How can you protect the client's scalp from burns while removing a curl from a thermal iron? _____

_____

128. The _____ curl is a method of curling hair by winding a strand around the rod.

129. The spiral curl creates hanging curls suitable for hairstyles that are:

_____ a) Short

_____ b) Medium

_____ c) Long

_____ d) Both medium and long

130. Describe how to create a spiral curl: _____

_____

_____

_____

_____

131. What are end curls? _____

_____

132. What factors determine whether end curls turn under or over? _____

_____

_____

133. _____ thermal iron curls are used to create volume or lift in a finished hairstyle.

134. What determines the type of volume curls to be used? _____

_____

135. Match each of the following base curl types with the volume it provides.

_____ Volume-base   a) Moderate

_____ Full-base   b) Slight

_____ Half-base   c) Maximum

_____ Off-base   d) Full

136. Why do volume-base curls provide maximum lift or volume? _____

_____

_____

137. How is a volume-base curl wound? _____

_____

_____

_____

_____

138. Explain how to wind full-base curls. _____

_____

_____

_____

_____

139. What kind of a curl can you expect to get with a half-base curl? _____

_____

140. Outline the procedure for winding a half-base curl. _____

_____

_____

_____

_____

141. A(n) _____ curl is placed completely off its base and offers a curl option with only slight lift or volume.

142. When a hairstyle is to finished with curls, brush the _____ curls last.

143. _____ combs cannot be used in thermal curling, because they are flammable.

144. Allowing hair ends to protrude over a thermal iron causes _____, hair that is bent or folded.

THERMAL HAIR STRAIGHTENING (HAIR PRESSING)

145. When done properly, _____ temporarily straightens extremely curly or unruly hair by means of a heated iron or comb.

146. How long does a pressing last? _____

_____

147. What additional services can hair pressing prepare the hair for? _____

_____

_____

148. A good hair pressing leaves the hair in a(n) _____ condition.

149. Match each of the following pressing types with the percentage of curl it removes from hair.

_____ Soft   a) 60 to 75

_____ Medium   b) 100

_____ Hard   c) 50 to 60

150. A(n) _____ press is accomplished by applying a thermal pressing comb once on each side of the hair.

151. A hard press, which involves applying a thermal pressing comb _____ on each side of the hair, is also called a(n) _____ press.

152. Before pressing a client's hair, analyze the condition of the _____ and _____.

153. When a client's hair and scalp are unhealthy, what should you do? _____

_____

_____

154. Failure to correct _____ hair can cause hair breakage during hair pressing.

155. What two things must you check before agreeing to give a pressing? _____

_____

156. A careful analysis of a client's hair should cover what points?

a) _____

b) _____

c) _____

d) _____

e) _____

f) _____

g) _____

h) _____

157. Why is it important for the cosmetologist to be able to recognize individual differences in hair texture, porosity, elasticity, and scalp flexibility? _____

_____

_____

_____

_____

158. Variations in hair texture have to do with the _____ of the hair and the _____ of the hair.

159. Coarse, extremely curly hair requires less heat and pressure than medium or fine hair in the pressing process.

_____ True

_____ False

160. Medium curly hair is the most resistant to hair pressing.

_____ True

_____ False

161. To avoid breaking fine hair, apply less heat and pressure than for other hair textures.

_____ True

_____ False

162. Which hair texture has qualities that make it difficult to press? _____

_____

163. What does wiry, curly hair feel like? _____

_____

164. What makes wiry hair resist hair pressing? _____

_____

165. Wiry hair requires _____ heat and pressure than other types of hair.

166. List the three possible conditions of a client's scalp.

a) _____

b) _____

c) _____

167. If the scalp is tight and the hair coarse, how should you press the hair?

_____

168. What should the cosmetologist remember with a flexible scalp? _____

_____

_____

169. During the client consultation, the cosmetologist should ask the client about which of the following?

_____ a) Lightener

_____ b) Tint

_____ c) Color restorer

_____ d) All of these answers are correct.

170. As with all services, the client should sign a(n) _____ before hair pressing to protect the school, the salon, and the stylist from liability due to accidents or damage.

171. The application of a conditioning treatment usually _____ hair pressing.

172. Explain how to make a tight scalp more flexible. _____

_____

173. What are the two types of pressing combs? _____

_____

174. What should pressing combs be made of? _____

_____

175. A pressing comb with little space between its teeth produces a _____ press.

176. Pressing combs are all the same size.

_____ True

_____ False

177. Why should you temper a new pressing comb made of brass? _____

_____

_____

178. How should you temper a new pressing comb? _____

_____

_____

179. When a pressing comb is being heated in a gas stove, its teeth should point _____ and the handle should be kept _____ from the fire.

180. How will you know when a pressing comb is too hot? _____

_____

181. Electric pressing combs are available in what two forms?

a) _____

b) _____

182. Describe how to clean a pressing comb: _____

_____

183. How can you remove carbon from a pressing comb? _____

_____

_____

_____

184. List the benefits of pressing oil or cream.

a) _____

b) _____

c) _____

d) _____

e) _____

f) _____

g) _____

185. When is a hard press recommended? _____

_____

186. A hard press is also known as a(n) _____ press.

187. What may cause pressed hair to curl again? _____

_____

188. The cosmetologist can prevent the smoking or burning of hair during a pressing treatment by _____

_____.

189. In the event of an accidental burn during pressing, what should you do immediately? _____

_____

190. When pressing coarse hair, apply enough pressure so that the hair remains

_____.

191. When pressing lightened or tinted hair, the client may need _____

_____.

192. Because gray hair may resist pressing, use a _____ pressing comb applied with _____ pressure.

STYLING LONG HAIR

193. Describe an updo: _____

_____

_____

194. Name three classic updo techniques.

a) _____

b) _____

c) _____

195. Identify the main sections of the pre-service procedure.

a) _____

b) _____

c) _____

d) _____

196. Outline the main steps of the post-service procedure.

a) _____

b) _____

c) _____

197. Explain how to find a client's natural part when preparing hair for wet styling.

_____

_____

_____

198. List the implements and materials needed for wet hairstyling.

a) _____

b) _____

c) _____

d) _____

e) _____

199. Describe the action in the illustrations below:

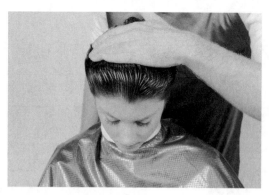 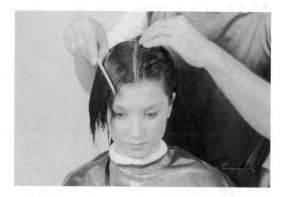

_____

200. Describe how to create a part:

a) _____

b) _____

c) _____

_____

201. List the implements and materials needed for horizontal finger waving.

a) _____

b) _____

c) _____

d) _____

e) _____

f) _____

g) _____

h) _____

i) _____

j) _____

202. How should you apply waving lotion during horizontal finger waving? _____

_____

_____

203. Horizontal finger waving should begin where?

_____ a) Forehead

_____ b) Hairline

_____ c) Nape

_____ d) Ear

204. To form the first ridge during horizontal finger waving, point the teeth of the comb _____.

205. In horizontal finger waving, the first and second ridges are created using the same movements.

_____ True

_____ False

206. Once an entire head is finger waved, what should you do? _____

_____

_____

_____

_____

207. How do you achieve a retro look upon finishing horizontal finger waving?

_____

_____

208. What does the accompanying figure illustrate? _____

_____

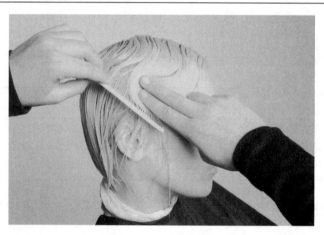

209. List the implements and materials needed for carved or sculpted curls.

a) _____

b) _____

c) _____

d) _____

e) _____

f) _____

g) _____

h) _____

i) _____

210. Describe how to make carved or sculpted curls after the first shaping:

a) _____

b) _____

c) _____

d) _____

211. Describe how to anchor a carved or sculpted curl:

a) _____

b) _____

c) _____

_____

d) _____

_____

212. How can you avoid an indentation or dent in a carved or sculpted curl?

_____

_____

213. What does the accompanying figure illustrate? _____

_____

214. What implements and materials are needed for a wet set with rollers?

a) _____

b) _____

c) _____

d) _____

e) _____

f) _____

g) _____

h) _____

i) _____

j) _____

215. To begin the wet set, you should _____

_____.

216. Begin setting wet rollers at the _____, parting off a section the same length and width as the roller.

217. In a wet set with rollers, what factor determines what type of base to use?

_____

_____

218. Loose rollers result in weak sets.

_____ True

_____ False

219. List the implements and materials needed for hair wrapping.

a) _____

b) _____

c) _____

d) _____

e) _____

f) _____

220. What product is appropriate for wrapping dry hair? _____

_____

_____

221. During hair wrapping, where should the hand rest to hold the head still?

_____

222. During hair wrapping, use a comb or brush in a(n) _____ motion to wrap the hair on the outer perimeter of the head in a(n) _____ direction.

223. While wrapping, use _____ to keep the hair in place.

224. Once all the hair is wrapped, you should _____

_____

_____ .

225. When working on dry hair, leave the hair wrapped for about _____ minutes.

226. When wrapping wet hair, place the client under a hooded dryer until the hair is completely dry, usually _____ minutes, depending on _____ .

227. List the implements and materials needed for blowdry styling.

a) _____

b) _____

c) _____

d) _____

e) _____

f) _____

g) _____

h) _____

228. List the steps to blowdry short, layered, curly hair to produce a smooth and full finish once a clean neck strip is in place.

a) _____

_____

b) _____

c) _____

_____

_____

d) _____

e) _____

_____

f) _____

229. When blowdrying hair, the hot air should flow _____

_____.

230. List the steps to blowdry short, curly hair in its natural wave pattern once liquid gel is applied.

a) _____

b) _____

_____

c) _____

_____

d) _____

_____

e) _____

_____

_____

_____

f) _____

231. List the steps to diffuse long, curly, or extremely curly hair in its natural wave pattern once a clean neck strip is in place.

a) _____

_____

b) _____

c) _____

_____

_____

232. List the steps to blowdry straight or wavy hair with maximum volume once a clean neck strip is in place.

a) _____

b) _____

_____

c) _____

_____

d) _____

_____

_____

e) _____

_____

f) _____

_____

233. What does the accompanying figure illustrate? _____

_____

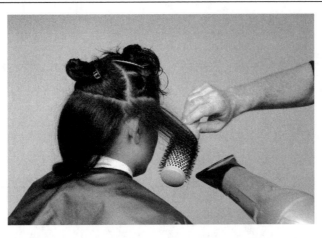

234. List the steps to blowdry blunt or long-layered, straight to wavy hair into a smooth straight style once gel is applied.

a) _____

_____

b) _____

_____

_____

c) _____

_____

_____

_____

_____

d) _____

_____

_____

e) _____

_____

_____

f) _____

_____

_____

_____

_____

g) _____

_____

_____

_____

h) _____

_____

_____

_____

_____

235. What does the accompanying figure illustrate? _____

_____

_____

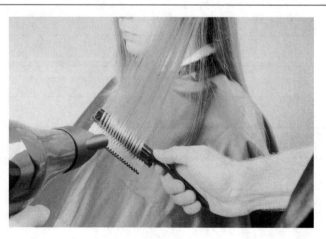

236. List the implements and materials needed for thermal waving.

a) _____

b) _____

c) _____

d) _____

237. In thermal waving, what factor determines whether the first wave is left-moving or right-moving? _____

_____

238. During thermal waving, how much hair should you insert into the iron at once?

_____

_____

239. Where should the groove of the iron be when you insert it into the hair?

_____

240. Once an iron is in hair, what should you do? _____

_____

_____

241. What does the accompanying figure illustrate? _____

_____

242. When curling short hair, the first section should be about _____ -inches (cm) wide and extend from the center of the _____ to the _____.

243. When curling short hair, the curl base is usually about 1½- to 2-inches (3.75 to 5 cm) wide.

_____ True

_____ False

244. What does the accompanying figure illustrate? _____

_____

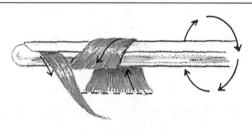

245. To curl medium length hair, you insert the hair into the open iron at the

_____.

246. Once the iron is in position to curl medium length hair, hold for about
_____ to heat the hair, and then slide it upward to _____
inch(es) (cm) from the scalp.

247. What does the accompanying figure illustrate? _____

_____

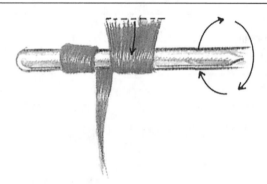

248. When curling hair using two loops or Figure 8, insert the hair into the open iron
about _____ inch(es) from the scalp.

_____ a) ¼

_____ b) ½

_____ c) 1

_____ d) 2

249. When curling hair using two loops or Figure 8, you pull the hair over the rod in
which direction? _____

_____

250. Use _____ tension when holding a strand of hair while curling using two
loops or Figure 8.

251. In what direction should you roll the iron when curling hair using two loops or Figure 8?

_____ a) Over

_____ b) Under

_____ c) Left

_____ d) Right

252. Describe how to even the distribution of hair when using two loops or Figure 8:

_____

_____

253. List the implements and materials needed to soft press normal curly hair.

a) _____

b) _____

c) _____

d) _____

e) _____

f) _____

g) _____

h) _____

i) _____

j) _____

k) _____

254. When soft pressing for normal curly hair, blowdrying leaves hair more manageable than hood drying.

_____ True

_____ False

255. When soft pressing for normal curly hair, divide the hair into _____ main sections.

256. For coarse hair with greater density, use _____ sections when soft pressing to ensure _____.

257. Before applying a heated pressing comb to hair, you should _____

_____.

258. When soft pressing for normal curly hair, what part of the comb actually does the pressing? _____

_____

259. Once you have soft pressed all normal curly hair, what do you apply? _____

_____

_____

260. List the implements and materials needed to style a knot or chignon.

a) _____

b) _____

c) _____

d) _____

e) _____

f) _____

g) _____

h) _____

i) _____

j) _____

k) _____

261. How should you secure the ponytail of a knot or chignon? _____

_____

_____

262. Explain how to conceal the elastic band of a knot or chignon. _____

_____

_____

263. How should you secure the underside of the roll? _____

264. List the steps to create a twist after the hair is blowdried.

a) _____

b) _____

_____

c) _____

_____

_____

d) _____

_____

_____

_____

e) _____

f) _____

_____

_____

_____

_____

265. For a pleat, you begin pinning the hair _____.

266. What does the accompanying figure illustrate? _____

_____

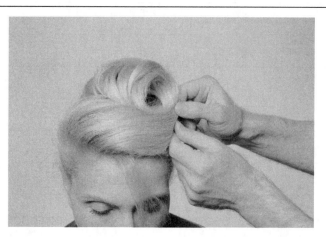

267. How should you finish a pleat? _____

_____

_____

18 Braiding and Braid Extensions

Date: _____

Rating: _____

Text Pages: 506–537

POINT TO PONDER:

"Life is like riding in a taxi. Whether you are going anywhere or not, the meter keeps ticking."—**John C. Maxwell**

WHY STUDY BRAIDING AND BRAID EXTENSIONS?

1. In your own words, explain why cosmetologists should thoroughly understand the importance of braiding and braid extensions.

_____

_____

_____

_____

_____

_____

_____

_____

2. Historically, the first highly decorative braids were seen among _____ tribes.

3. Today, braids are as acceptable as any other hairstyle in most modern workplaces.

_____ True

_____ False

4. Braiding salons practice what is commonly known as _____ hairstyling, which uses no chemicals or dyes and does not alter the natural curl or coil pattern of the hair.

5. With proper care, a braided hair design can last up to ____ months, with ____ to ____ weeks being preferable.

6. What is the best way to avoid misunderstandings and ensure a happy ending to every natural-styling service? _____

_____

_____

UNDERSTANDING THE BASICS

7. When analyzing the condition of a client's hair and scalp during consultation, you should pay particular attention to the hair's _____.

8. In braiding and other natural hairstyling, texture refers to what three qualities?

   a) _____

   b) _____

   c) _____

9. In addition to texture, the cosmetologist should consider what characteristics during hair analysis?

   a) _____

   b) _____

   c) _____

   d) _____

10. Everyone has thinner, finer hair around the hairline.

   _____ True

   _____ False

11. In the natural hairstyling/braiding world, hair is referred to as _____ or _____ when it has had no chemical treatments.

12. _____ involves overlapping two strands of hair to achieve a candy cane effect.

13. Interweaving a weft or faux hair with natural hair is known as _____.

14. Some states have separate natural hairstyling licenses.

   _____ True

   _____ False

15. Stylists who hold only braiding, natural hairstyling, or locktician licenses can perform such chemical services as coloring or perming.

_____ True

_____ False

16. Identify the tools used for braiding:

a) _____

b) _____

c) _____

d) _____

e) _____

f) _____

g) _____

h) _____

i) _____

j) _____

k) _____

l) _____

m) _____

n) _____

o) _____

p) _____

17. What is the advantage of using a boar-bristle brush? _____

_____

_____

18. Explain the use of the square paddle brush in braiding. _____

_____

_____

_____

_____

_____

19. In braiding, the vent brush is used to _____

_____ .

20. The distance between teeth is the most important feature of a wide-toothed comb.

_____ True

_____ False

21. Which of the following tools is excellent for design parting, sectioning large segments of hair, and opening and removing braids?

_____ a) Diffuser

_____ b) Long clip

_____ c) Tail comb

_____ d) Finishing comb

22. Identify the implements and materials needed for extensions:

a) _____

b) _____

c) _____

23. What is a hackle? _____

_____

_____

24. A(n) _____ is a flat leather pad with very close, fine teeth that sandwiches human hair extensions.

25. The fibers used largely determine an extension's success and durability.

_____ True

_____ False

26. List some materials commonly used for hair extensions.

a) _____

b) _____

c) _____

d) _____

e) _____

f) _____

27. What is Kanekalon, and why is it a good choice for extensions?

_____

_____

_____

_____

28. Discuss the pros and cons of nylon or rayon synthetic. _____

_____

_____

_____

_____

_____

29. Why is traditional yarn now being used to adorn hair? _____

_____

_____

_____

_____

30. Why should care be taken when purchasing yarn? _____

_____

_____

31. _____, a beautiful wool fiber imported from Africa, has a matte finish and comes only in black and brown.

32. The strong fiber that comes from the domestic ox found in the mountains of Tibet and Central Asia is _____.

33. Why is it best to braid curly hair when it is dry? _____

_____

_____

_____

34. Straight, resistant hair is best braided slightly damp or very lightly coated with a(n) _____ or _____ to make it more pliable.

35. Textured hair is very fragile both wet and dry.

_____ True

_____ False

36. List the steps in the cleaning and disinfecting portion of the pre-service procedure.

a) _____

b) _____

_____

_____

c) _____

_____

_____

d) _____

_____

e) _____

f) _____

g) _____

_____

37. What questions should the stylist ask to help prepare the client for a positive experience?

a) _____

b) _____

c) _____

_____

d) _____

_____

e) _____

f) _____

_____

38. What are the three main task areas of the post-service procedure?

a) _____

b) _____

c) _____

39. List all of the implements, materials, and supplies needed to prepare textured hair for braiding.

a) _____

b) _____

c) _____

d) _____

e) _____

f) _____

g) _____

h) _____

i) _____

40. When preparing textured hair for braiding, part the back of the head into _____ to _____ sections. For thick, textured hair, make _____ sections; for thinner hair, user _____ sections.

41. Explain how to blowdry textured hair as part of the pre-service procedure.

_____

_____

_____

_____

_____

_____

BRAIDING THE HAIR

42. A(n) _____ braid is a three-stand braid created with a(n) _____ technique in which the left section goes under the middle strand, then the right section goes under the middle strand.

43. A(n) _____ or _____ braid is a three-strand braid produced with a(n) _____ technique in which the first side section goes over the middle one, then the other side section goes over the middle strand.

44. What type of braid is made with two strands twisted around each other?

_____

45. Outline the procedure for creating a rope braid.

a) _____

b) _____

c) _____

d) _____

_____

e) _____

_____

f) _____

_____

g) _____

h) _____

_____

i) _____

_____

j) _____

k) _____

_____

l) _____

_____

m) _____

_____

n) _____

_____

_____

_____

o) _____

_____

46. The _____ braid is a simple, two-strand braid in which hair is picked up from the sides and added to the strands as they are crossed over each other.

47. The fishtail braid is best done on layered hair that is less than shoulder length.

_____ True

_____ False

48. What does the accompanying figure illustrate? _____

_____

49. The invisible braid is ideal for long hair but can be executed on shorter hair with long layers.

_____ True

_____ False

50. To begin the procedure for an invisible braid, start at the _____ of the head, take a(n) _____ section of hair, and place it in your _____ hand. Divide the section into _____ equal strands, _____ in the left hand and _____ in the right.

51. What do the terms single braids, box braids, and individual braids refer to?

_____

_____

_____

52. The partings or subsections for single braids can be what shape?

a) _____

b) _____

c) _____

53. With single braids, the _____ determines where the braid is placed and how it moves.

54. Extensions for single braids come in a wide range of sizes and lengths and are integrated into the natural hair using the _____ technique.

55. Fiber for extensions can be selected from _____, _____, or _____.

56. Discuss the process for preparing a client for a single braid. _____

_____

_____

_____

_____

_____

_____

_____

57. What is the procedure for creating a single braid without extensions?

a) _____

b) _____

c) _____

d) _____

_____

e) _____

_____

f) _____

_____

g) _____

_____

h) _____

_____

_____

i) _____

_____

j) _____

_____

_____

k) _____

_____

l) _____

m) _____

_____

n) _____

_____

58. What portion of the procedure for single braid with extension does the accompanying figure illustrate? _____

_____

_____

59. _____, also called _____, are narrow rows of visible braids that lie close to the scalp.

60. How are cornrows created? _____

_____

61. How long do cornrows last? _____

_____

_____

62. Explain why the feed-in method is used for cornrows with extensions. _____

_____

_____

_____

_____

_____

63. Compare traditional cornrows with those created with the feed-in method.

_____

_____

_____

_____

_____

_____

64. Give some options for finishing basic cornrows. _____

_____

_____

_____

65. Outline the procedure for creating cornrows with extensions.

a) _____

b) _____

c) _____

d) _____

_____

e) _____

_____

_____

_____

f) _____

g) _____

_____

_____

h) _____

_____

_____

_____

_____

i) _____

66. Discuss the technique of tree braiding and how they are created. _____

_____

_____

_____

_____

_____

_____

_____

67. What are hair locks? _____

_____

68. List and briefly explain the three basic methods of locking.

a) _____

_____

b) _____

_____

c) _____

_____

CHAPTER 19 Wigs and Hair Additions

Date: _____

Rating: _____

Text Pages: 538–561

POINT TO PONDER:

"There are two types of people who never achieve much in their lifetime. The person who won't do what he is told, and the person who does no more than he is told."—**Andrew Carnegie**

1. The _____ shaved their heads with bronze razors and wore heavy black wigs to protect themselves from the sun.

2. In ancient _____, women wore wigs made from the prized blond hair of barbarians captured from the north.

3. In eighteenth-century England, men wore wigs, called _____, to indicate that they were in the army or navy or engaged in the practice of law.

4. Most clients today have their wigs custom fitted.

   _____ True

   _____ False

5. Toupees are often custom made and fitted.

   _____ True

   _____ False

WHY STUDY WIGS AND HAIR ADDITIONS?

6. In your own words, explain why cosmetologists should study and thoroughly understand wigs and hair additions._____

   _____

   _____

   _____

   _____

   _____

   _____

_____

_____

HUMAN VERSUS SYNTHETIC HAIR

7. Describe the fastest way to tell if a hair strand is synthetic or human:_____

_____

_____

_____

_____

_____

8. List the advantages of human hair.

a) _____

b) _____

c) _____

9. List the disadvantages of human hair.

a) _____

b) _____

c) _____

d) _____

10. List the advantages of synthetic hair.

a) _____

b) _____

c) _____

d) _____

e) _____

f) _____

g) _____

h) _____

i) _____

11. List the disadvantages of synthetic hair.

a) _____

b) _____

c) _____

d) _____

12. The most expensive wigs, hairpieces, and extensions are made of human hair.

_____ True

_____ False

13. Top-of-the-line wigs are made of European hair.

_____ True

_____ False

14. Color-treated hair is the most costly.

_____ True

_____ False

15. What two regions of the world provide most commercial human hair?

_____ a) India and South America

_____ b) Middle East and India

_____ c) Asia and North America

_____ d) India and Asia

16. Indian hair is usually available in lengths from _____ to _____ inches.

_____ a) 3 to 7

_____ b) 8 to 12

_____ c) 12 to 16

_____ d) 12 to 28

17. Asian hair is available in lengths from _____ to _____ inches.

_____ a) 3 to 7

_____ b) 8 to 12

_____ c) 12 to 16

_____ d) 12 to 28

18. Indian hair is naturally _____, whereas Asian hair is naturally _____.

19. Is human hair ever mixed with other fibers in wigs? If so, what kind? _____

_____

_____

20. Mixed-hair products are used most often for which of the following?

_____ a) Hair competitions

_____ b) Cancer patients

_____ c) Theatrical settings

_____ d) Bridal updos

21. What questions should you ask when selecting a hair addition for a client?

a) _____

_____

b) _____

c) _____

d) _____

e) _____

f) _____

g) _____

_____

h) _____

i) _____

j) _____

22. What is turned hair? _____

_____

_____

23. Define the term fallen hair. _____

_____

_____

_____

WIGS

24. A(n) _____ can be defined as an artificial covering for the head consisting of a network of interwoven hair.

25. If a hair addition does not fully cover the head, it is either a(n) _____, which is a small wig used to cover the top or crown of the head, or a hair _____ of some sort.

26. Name the two basic categories of wigs.

    a) _____

    b) _____

27. _____ wigs are constructed with an elasticized mesh-fiber base to which the hair is attached.

28. How are cap wigs sized? _____

    _____

29. What does it mean if a cap wig is hand-knotted? _____

    _____

30. How are cap wigs fitted to the head? _____

    _____

    _____

    _____

31. _____ wigs are machine-made from human or artificial hair.

32. Long strips of hair with a threaded edge are known as _____.

33. Why are capless wigs more popular than cap wigs? _____

    _____

34. Capless wigs are extremely light and comfortable to wear due to their _____ and _____.

35. What type of client is a cap wig best suited for, and why? _____

    _____

    _____

36. Match each of the following wigs with its description.

_____ 1. Hand-tied or hand-knotted wig

a) Made by feeding wefts through a sewing machine and then sewing them together to form the wig's base and shape

_____ 2. Semi-hand-tied wig

b) Made by inserting individual strands of hair into a mesh foundation and knotting them with a needle

_____ 3. Machine-made wig

c) Constructed with a combination of synthetic hair and hand-tied human hair

37. Explain why is it important to note the artificial growth patterns of a wig.

_____

_____

38. The most flexible and versatile of all patterns is the _____ wig.

39. _____ wigs are sewn in an exact direction, offering no versatility.

40. The creation of a custom-made wig begins with _____

_____.

41. Most wig manufacturers ask for precise specifications of what characteristics?

a) _____

b) _____

c) _____

d) _____

42. Why do ready-to-wear wigs require no measuring? _____

_____

_____

43. No matter what type of wig is used, every wig needs to be adjusted to the head and _____ to suit the client.

44. A(n) _____ is a head-shaped form, usually made of canvas-covered cork or Styrofoam, on which the wig is secured for fitting, coloring, and sometimes styling.

45. The block is best attached to the work area with a swivel clamp.

_____ True

_____ False

46. Most wigs today are cleaned while on the client.

_____ True

_____ False

47. Describe the proper procedure for putting on a wig: _____

_____

_____

_____

_____

_____

48. What implements and material will you need in order to measure a client for a custom-made wig?

49. When cutting a wig, generally the goal is to _____.

50. When cutting and trimming wigs, what basic methods of haircutting should you follow? _____

_____

_____

51. When free-form cutting, vertical sections create _____, diagonal sections create a(n) _____ edge, and horizontal sections build _____.

52. Free-form cutting is usually done on dry hair, which allows you to see more easily how the hair will fall.

_____ True

_____ False

53. Compare the wet cutting method with the dry cutting method. _____

_____

_____

54. A more abstract cutting method often results in a cut that looks less realistic.

_____ True

_____ False

55. When using heat on a human-hair wig, always set the styling tool to what position?

_____ Low

_____ Medium

_____ High

56. Traditionally, brushes made with _____ have been regarded as best for use on human hair.

57. Comb-outs and finishing touches for most modern cuts should be done on the block.

_____ True

_____ False

58. For a wig to look believable, what areas must appear the most convincing?

a) _____

b) _____

c) _____

59. To style a wig to look as natural as possible always follow the direction of the

_____.

60. What type of styling products should be used on a human-hair wig? _____

_____

_____

61. To make the hairline of a wig look natural, you should _____ gently around the hairline.

62. What is a wind test? _____

_____

_____

63. When styling a wig, you should make the final results look perfect.

_____ True

_____ False

64. What is the best way to clean any wig? _____

_____

_____

_____

_____

_____

65. Most commercially available wigs are what colors? _____

_____

_____

66. If you are going to custom-color wig hair, use hair that has been decolorized through the _____ , process not with _____ dyes.

67. The first step when coloring a wig is to _____ .

68. Hair in which the cuticle is absent is very _____ and will react to color in an extreme manner.

69. Always _____ test hair before a full-color application.

70. When coloring a wig, what color products can be used?

a) _____

b) _____

c) _____

d) _____

e) _____

71. When coloring a human-hair wig or hairpiece, conduct regular color checks every _____ to _____ minutes.

72. Often, it is easier to color a client's hair to match a hair addition than to color the addition itself.

_____ True

_____ False

If you want to perm human hair to match a client's natural wave pattern, you must know how the hair was colored.

_____ True

_____ False

73. You may safely perm wig hair that has been colored with a metallic dye.

_____ True

_____ False

74. Where should an addition be while performing a permanent wave?

_____

_____

_____

HAIRPIECES

75. What is a hairpiece, and how much coverage does it give? _____

_____

_____

76. List some different types of hairpieces.

a) _____

b) _____

c) _____

77. A(n) _____ hairpiece has openings in the base through which the client's own hair is pulled to blend with the natural or synthetic hair of the hairpiece.

78. Hairpieces are very lightweight, natural-looking products that add _____ and _____ to the client's hair.

79. A(n) _____ is a small wig used to cover the top and crown of the head.

80. What are the two ways to attach toupees?

a) _____

b) _____

81. _____ hairpieces, which include things like ponytails, chignons, and cascades, are a great salon product for special occasions or for use as fashion accessories.

82. Fashion hairpieces vary in _____ and are constructed on a _____.

83. Identify some temporary means for attaching fashion hairpieces:

a) _____

b) _____

c) _____

d) _____

e) _____

HAIR EXTENSIONS

84. _____ are hair additions that are secured to the base of the client's natural hair to add length, volume, texture, or color.

85. What general guidelines should you keep in mind when attaching hair extensions?

a) _____

b) _____

_____

c) _____

_____

d) _____

e) _____

_____

f) _____

86. Name some ways to attach hair additions.

a) _____

b) _____

c) _____

d) _____

87. The most important professional approaches to hair addition and extension services should be practiced in the following order:

a) _____

b) _____

c) _____

d) _____

88. In the _____, hair extensions are secured to the client's own hair by sewing braids or a weft onto an on-the-scalp braid or cornrow, sometimes called the _____.

89. In the braid-and-sew method, the _____ of the track determines how the hair will fall.

90. Identify the directions in which tracks positioned in the braid-and-sew method:

a) _____

b) _____

c) _____

d) _____

91. In the braid-and-sew method, it is best to place the tracks or braids _____ inch(es) (cm) behind the hairline to ensure proper coverage.

92. How are extensions sewn onto a track in the braid-and-sew method?

_____

_____

_____

93. Name the stitches that may be used to sew extensions to a track.

a) _____

b) _____

c) _____

94. _____ involves attaching hair wefts or single strands with an adhesive or bonding agent.

95. Generally, bonding product will last from _____ to _____ weeks.

96. What factors affect how long hair will remain bonded?

a) _____

b) _____

c) _____

97. Describe the bonding procedure, step-by-step:

a) _____

b) _____

_____

c) _____

d) _____

e) _____

_____

f) _____

g) _____

_____

98. Discuss the advantages of bonding. _____

_____

_____

_____

99. In the _____ method of attaching extensions, extension hair is bonded to the client's own hair with a bonding material that is activated by the heat from a special tool.

100. What are the advantages of the fusion method?

a) _____

_____

b) _____

c) _____

101. How long do fused attachments last? _____

_____

102. What does the accompanying figure depict? _____

_____

_____

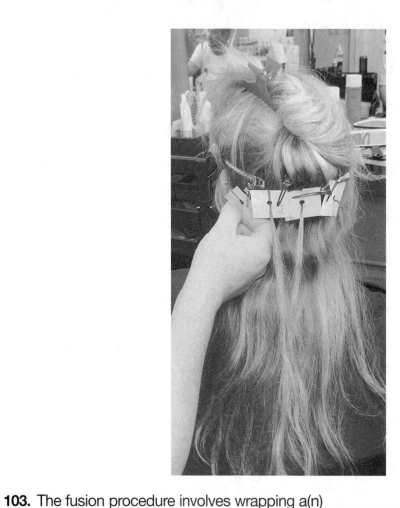

103. The fusion procedure involves wrapping a(n) _____ strip around both the client's hair and the extension.

104. Discuss the drawbacks of fusion bonding. _____

_____

_____

_____

_____

_____

105. Give an overview of the linking process. _____

_____

_____

_____

_____

_____

106. Generally, the problems with tube shrinking arise from the materials, not the stylist.

_____ True

_____ False

107. What are some guidelines for retailing hair goods or offering hair-addition services?

a) _____

b) _____

c) _____

d) _____

e) _____

f) _____

g) _____

_____

20 Chemical Texture Services

Date: _____

Rating: _____

Text Pages: 562–625

POINT TO PONDER:

"Nothing great was ever achieved without enthusiasm."
—Ralph Waldo Emerson

WHY STUDY CHEMICAL TEXTURE SERVICES?

1. In your own words, explain why cosmetologists should study and thoroughly understand chemical texture services. _____

_____

_____

_____

_____

_____

_____

_____

_____

2. _____ are hair services that cause chemical changes that alter the hair's natural wave pattern

3. Identify some chemical texture services:

a) _____

b) _____

c) _____

THE STRUCTURE OF HAIR

4. Name the layers of the hair.

a) _____

b) _____

c) _____

5. The cuticle is directly involved in the texture or movement of the hair.

_____ True

_____ False

6. The medulla plays no role in chemical texture services and may be missing in fine hair.

_____ True

_____ False

7. The natural pH of hair is between _____ and _____.

8. Chemical texturizers _____ the pH of the hair to an alkaline state to soften and swell the hair shaft.

9. Coarse, resistant hair with a strong, compact cuticle layer requires a highly alkaline chemical solution.

_____ True

_____ False

10. List the basic building blocks of hair.

a) _____

b) _____

c) _____

d) _____

e) _____

11. _____ bonds, also known as end bonds, are chemical bonds that join amino acids, end-to-end in long chains, to form a polypeptide chain.

12. Side bonds are _____, _____, and _____ bonds that cross-link polypeptide chains.

13. Disulfide bonds can be broken by the extreme heat produced by some thermal styling tools.

_____ True

_____ False

14. Disulfide bonds are the weakest of the three side bonds.

_____ True

_____ False

15. Salt bonds are broken by changes in pH.

_____ True

_____ False

16. Individual hydrogen bonds are very weak.

_____ True

_____ False

PERMANENT WAVING

17. _____ is a two-step process in which the hair undergoes a physical change caused by wrapping the hair on perm rods and then causing a chemical change by applying permanent waving solution and neutralizer.

18. You should always perform an elasticity test before perming the hair.

_____ True

_____ False

19. A wet set breaks _____ bonds, whereas a permanent wave breaks _____ bonds.

20. In permanent waving, what two factors determine curl size?

a) _____

b) _____

21. List the types of rods used in chemical texture services.

a) _____

b) _____

c) _____

d) _____

22. _____ rods produce a tighter curl in the center and a looser curl on either side of the strand.

23. Soft bender rods are usually about _____ -inches (cm) long with a uniform diameter along the entire length.

24. End papers should extend beyond the ends of the hair to prevent _____, hair that is bent up at the ends.

25. Name the most common end paper techniques.

a) _____

b) _____

c) _____

26. What is the purpose of the double flat wrap? _____

_____

_____

27. The _____ wrap eliminates excess paper and can be used with short rods or with very short lengths of hair.

28. _____ are subsections of panels into which the hair is divided for perm wrapping.

29. Explain how base placement is determined. _____

_____

30. Using a base section that is wider than the perm rod can create an uneven curl pattern and undue tension on the hair.

_____ True

_____ False

31. In which type of base placement is the hair wrapped at a 90-degree angle?

_____ a) On base

_____ b) Half off base

_____ c) Off base

_____ d) All answers are correct.

32. _____ refers to the angle at which the rod is positioned on the head.

33. A(n) _____ wrap is wrapped from the ends to the scalp in overlapping concentric layers.

34. In a spiral perm wrap, the hair is wrapped perpendicular to the length of the rod.

_____ True

_____ False

35. Alkaline permanent waving solutions soften and swell the hair.

_____ True

_____ False

36. Name the reactions that occur in the chemical process of permanent waving.

a) _____

b) _____

_____

c) _____

_____

d) _____

_____

37. All permanent wave solutions contain a reducing agent.

_____ True

_____ False

38. _____, a colorless liquid with a strong, unpleasant odor, is the most common reducing agent in permanent wave solutions.

39. The alkalinity of the perm solution should correspond to the _____, _____, and _____ of the cuticle layer.

40. Alkaline waves have a pH between _____ and _____.

41. _____ is the main active ingredient in true acid and acid-balanced waving lotions.

42. List the three components of all acid waves.

a) _____

b) _____

c) _____

43. Explain how a true acid wave, with a pH below 7.0, can cause the hair to swell.

_____

_____

_____

_____

44. Pure water can damage the hair.

_____ True

_____ False

45. Discuss the effect of higher pH on acid-balanced waves. _____

_____

_____

_____

46. An exothermic chemical reaction absorbs heat.

_____ True

_____ False

47. Give two examples of alkanolamines that are used in permanent waving solutions as substitutes for ammonia.

a) _____

b) _____

48. Permanents based on sulfites are very weak and do not provide firm curls, especially on strong or resistant hair.

_____ True

_____ False

49. Hair that has been treated with semipermanent color is less porous than hair treated with permanent color.

_____ True

_____ False

50. Which of the following perm types is recommended for extremely porous hair?

_____ a) Alkaline/cold wave

_____ b) Thio-free wave

_____ c) True acid wave

_____ d) Exothermic wave

51. Explain how the strength and processing amount of a permanent wave process is determined. _____

_____

_____

52. _____ is essential to proper processing in all permanent waves.

53. A properly processed permanent wave should break and rebuild approximately _____ percent of the hair's disulfide bonds.

54. Overprocessed hair is overly curly.

_____ True

_____ False

55. Underprocessed hair is usually straighter at the scalp and curlier at the ends.

_____ True

_____ False

56. In permanent waving, _____ stops the action of the waving solution and rebuilds the hair into its new curly form.

57. Identify the two functions of neutralization:

a) _____

b) _____

58. The most common neutralizer is _____.

59. Give some tips for proper rinsing and blotting during thio neutralization.

a) _____

b) _____

c) _____

d) _____

e) _____

_____

f) _____

g) _____

_____

h) _____

_____

i) _____

_____

j) _____

_____

60. Identify the information preliminary test curls provide:

a) _____

b) _____

c) _____

_____

61. Give the steps for the stylist preparation portion of the pre-service procedure.

a) _____

_____

b) _____

_____

c) _____

_____

_____

_____

d) _____

_____

_____

e) _____

_____

_____

f) _____

62. Outline the portion of the post-service procedure dedicated to preparing the work area and implements for the next client.

a) _____

_____

_____

_____

b) _____

_____

c) _____

_____

63. Name the implements, materials, and supplies needed to perform a preliminary test curl for a permanent wave.

a) _____

b) _____

c) _____

d) _____

e) _____

f) _____

g) _____

h) _____

i) _____

j) _____

k) _____

l) _____

m) _____

n) _____

o) _____

p) _____

q) _____

r) _____

s) _____

t) _____

64. Specify the three basic wrapping patterns.

a) _____

b) _____

c) _____

65. The _____ is the position of the tool in relation to its base section, determined by the angle at which the hair is wrapped.

66. In the procedure for permanent wave and processing using a basic permanent wrap, you wrap the hair into _____ panels.

67. What is the proper procedure for wrapping panels in permanent wave and processing using a basic permanent wrap?

a) _____

_____

_____

b) _____

_____

_____

c) _____

_____

_____

68. Discuss the sectioning procedure for permanent wave and processing using a curvature permanent wrap._____

_____

_____

_____

_____

69. Outline the procedure for permanent wave and processing using a bricklay permanent wrap.

a) _____

_____

_____

_____

b) _____

c) _____

_____

_____

d) _____

_____

_____

_____

e) _____

_____

_____

_____

_____

f) _____

g) _____

_____

_____

h) _____

_____

_____

_____

i) _____

_____

_____

_____

j) _____

70. The _____ technique uses zigzag partings to divide base areas.

71. What is the procedure for permanent wave and processing using a weave technique?

a) _____

_____

_____

_____

b) _____

c) _____

_____

_____

d) _____

_____

_____

e) _____

_____

f) _____

_____

g) _____

_____

h) _____

_____

i) _____

72. What is the double-rod or piggyback wrap technique? _____

_____

_____

_____

_____

_____

_____

73. Name all the implements, materials, and supplies needed for permanent wave and processing using a spiral wrap technique.

a) _____

b) _____

c) _____

d) _____

e) _____

f) _____

g) _____

h) _____

i) _____

j) _____

k) _____

l) _____

m) _____

n) _____

o) _____

p) _____

q) _____

r) _____

s) _____

t) _____

74. Partial perms can be used for what kinds of clients?

a) _____

_____

b) _____

c) _____

_____

75. What additional considerations are there for partial perms?

a) _____

_____

b) _____

_____

_____

76. Why are many male clients requesting perms?

a) _____

b) _____

c) _____

d) _____

77. What problems can a perm help a male client with?

a) _____

b) _____

c) _____

78. The techniques for permanent waving men's hair differ from those used on women.

_____ True

_____ False

79. List the safety precautions for permanent waving.

a) _____

_____

_____

b) _____

_____

c) _____

_____

d) _____

e) _____

_____

f) _____

_____

g) _____

_____

h) _____

_____

i) _____

_____

j) _____

k) _____

l) _____

m) _____

_____

CHEMICAL HAIR RELAXERS

80. _____ is a process or service that rearranges the structure of curly hair into a straighter or smoother form.

81. What are the two most common types of chemical hair relaxers?

a) _____

b) _____

82. In extremely curly hair, the thinnest and weakest sections are at the twists.

_____ True

_____ False

83. _____ is the measurement of the thickness or thinness of a liquid that affects how the fluid flows.

84. Most relaxers contain the same ingredients used in depilatories.

_____ True

_____ False

85. The chemical reactions of thio relaxers differ from those used in permanent waving.

_____ True

_____ False

86. Explain how to avoid scalp irritation when applying thio relaxer to virgin hair._____

_____

87. Discuss the proper procedure for applying thio relaxer to virgin hair once protective base cream has been applied._____

_____

_____

_____

_____

_____

_____

_____

_____

_____

88. For a thio relaxer retouch, divide the hair into _____ sections.

89. Explain what to do during a thio relaxer retouch once the relaxer has been applied to all sections.

a) _____

_____

_____

_____

b) _____

_____

_____

_____

_____

c) _____

d) _____

_____

_____

_____

_____

_____

e) _____

f) _____

_____

g) _____

h) _____

90. What is the general procedure for Japanese thermal straighteners?

_____

_____

_____

_____

_____

_____

_____

_____

91. Hydroxide relaxers are compatible with thio relaxers, permanent waving, and soft curl perms.

_____ True

_____ False

92. The average pH of the hair is _____, and many hydroxide relaxers have a pH _____.

93. In _____, the process by which hydroxide relaxers permanently straighten hair, the relaxers remove a sulfur atom from a disulfide bond and convert it into a lanthionine bond.

94. Identify the types of hydroxide relaxers:

a) _____

b) _____

c) _____

95. What are the two most common low-pH relaxers?

a) _____

b) _____

96. _____, also known as protective base cream, is an oily cream used to protect the skin and scalp during hair relaxing.

97. Protective base cream should not touch the hair because it will slow the chemical straightening process.

_____ True

_____ False

98. Most chemical relaxers are available in what three strengths?

a) _____

b) _____

c) _____

99. All demipermanent haircoloring uses low volumes of peroxide or other alkalizing agents.

_____ True

_____ False

100. What is the purpose of periodic strand testing?_____

_____

101. Unlike thio neutralization, _____ is an acid-alkali neutralization that neutralizes (deactivates) the alkaline residues left in the hair by a hydroxide relaxer and lowers the pH of the hair and scalp.

102. Because the scalp area and porous hair ends usually process more quickly than the middle of the strand, the application for a virgin relaxer starts _____ to _____ inch(es) (cm) from the scalp.

103. What is the proper way to apply hydroxide relaxer to virgin hair? _____

_____

_____

_____

_____

_____

_____

104. What is the proper procedure when hair ends need additional relaxing during a hydroxide relaxer retouch? _____

_____

_____

_____

105. Which of the following relaxers is compatible with soft curl permanents?

_____ a) Guanidine hydroxide

_____ b) Ammonium thioglycolate

_____ c) Sodium hydroxide

_____ d) Lithium hydroxide

106. Keratin alone will straighten hair.

_____ True

_____ False

107. How do keratin straightening treatments work? _____

_____

_____

108. Preconditioning before a keratin straightening treatment is meant to _____

_____.

109. If a client wishes to have a demi-gloss treatment, it should be done at least ____ to ____ days after the keratin treatment.

CURL RE-FORMING (SOFT CURL PERMANENT)

110. A(n) _____ is a combination of a thio relaxer and a thio permanent that is wrapped on large rods to make existing curl larger and looser.

111. List the materials, implements, and supplies needed for curl re-forming (soft curl perm).

a) _____

b) _____

c) _____

d) _____

e) _____

f) _____

g) _____

h) _____

i) _____

j) _____

112. Give some safety precautions for hair relaxing and curl re-forming.

a) _____

_____

b) _____

_____

c) _____

_____

d) _____

_____

e) _____

_____

f) _____

_____

g) _____

h) _____

_____

i) _____

j) _____

_____

k) _____

l) _____

m) _____

n) _____

_____

o) _____

_____

p) _____

_____

q) _____

r) _____

_____

s) _____

_____

t) _____

u) _____

_____

v) _____

_____

w) _____

_____

x) _____

_____

y) _____

113. What is a curl re-forming? _____

_____

114. By what other name is a soft curl permanent called? _____

_____

115. What effect does a soft curl permanent have on the hair? _____

_____

116. List all the implements and supplies needed for a soft curl perm.

a) _____

b) _____

c) _____

d) _____

e) _____

f) _____

g) _____

h) _____

i) _____

j) _____

k) _____

l) _____

m) _____

n) _____

o) _____

p) _____

q) _____

r) _____

s) _____

t) _____

u) _____

v) _____

117. How do you prepare yourself and your client for a soft curl permanent?

a) _____

b) _____

c) _____

_____

d) _____

118. The first step in the soft curl permanent procedure is to follow the procedure for applying a _____.

119. After the hair has processed and is rinsed, part the hair into _____ panels.

120. Use the length of the _____ to measure the width of the panels.

121. Where should you begin wrapping? _____

122. Apply and distribute the thio curl booster to each _____ as you wrap.

123. What size should the horizontal partings be? _____

124. Hold the hair at a _____ angle to the head, roll the hair down to the scalp and position the rod _____.

125. Place cotton around the _____ and apply thio curl booster to all the curls until they are _____.

126. When processing is completed, rinse the hair thoroughly, for at least _____, and then towel-blot the hair on each rod to _____

_____.

127. Apply the _____ slowly and carefully to the hair on each rod.

128. Describe the clean-up procedure for this service:

a) _____

b) _____

c) _____

d) _____

e) _____

129. It is advisable to apply a hydroxide relaxer on hair that has been previously treated with a thio relaxer.

_____ True

_____ False

130. Do not apply a thio relaxer on hair that has been previously treated with a hydroxide relaxer.

_____ True

_____ False

131. Do not chemically relax hair that has been treated with a metallic dye.

_____ True

_____ False

132. It is advisable to shampoo the client's hair prior to the application of a hydroxide relaxer.

_____ True

_____ False

133. If any solution accidentally gets into a client's eye, _____

_____.

CHAPTER 21 Haircoloring

Date: _____

Rating: _____

Text Pages: 626–684

POINT TO PONDER:

"You can't depend on your judgment when your imagination is out of focus."—**Mark Twain**

1. Clients who have their hair colored usually visit the salon every _____ to _____ weeks.

WHY STUDY HAIRCOLORING?

2. In your own words, explain why cosmetologists should study and thoroughly understand hair coloring. _____

_____

_____

_____

_____

_____

_____

WHY PEOPLE COLOR THEIR HAIR

3. Identify the reasons people color their hair:

   a) _____

   b) _____

   c) _____

   d) _____

   e) _____

4. _____ is a professional, industry-coined term referring to artificial haircolor products and services, while _____ refers to the natural color of hair.

HAIR FACTS

5. The structure of the client's hair and the desired results determine which haircolor to use.

_____ True

_____ False

6. Name the three major components of hair.

a) _____

b) _____

c) _____

7. The _____, the middle layer of hair, gives the hair most of its strength and elasticity.

8. In hair, melanin is distributed differently according to texture.

_____ True

_____ False

9. Hair _____, the number of hairs per square inch (2.5 square cm), can range from thin to thick.

10. Define the term porosity. _____

11. In hair of _____ porosity, the cuticle is slightly raised.

12. Outline the procedure for testing for porosity.

a) _____

_____

b) _____

_____

c) _____

_____

_____

d) _____

e) _____

_____

IDENTIFYING NATURAL HAIR COLOR AND TONE

13. List the three types of melanin in the cortex.

a) _____

b) _____

c) _____

14. _____, also known as undertone, is the varying degrees of warmth exposed during a permanent color or lightening process.

15. _____ is the unit of measurement used to identify the lightness or darkness of a color.

16. Haircolor levels are arranged on a scale of 1 to 10, with ____ being the darkest and _____ the lightest.

17. Artificial light has no impact on the perception of color.

_____ True

_____ False

18. The first step when performing a haircolor service is to _____

_____.

19. What are the four steps to determining natural level?

a) _____

_____

b) _____

_____

_____

_____

c) _____

d) _____

20. A(n) _____ color is the predominant tone of a color.

21. Equal parts of blue and yellow always make green.

_____ True

_____ False

22. _____ colors are pure or fundamental colors (red, yellow, and blue) that cannot be created by combining other colors.

23. Which of the following is the weakest of the primary colors?

_____ a) Yellow

_____ b) Blue

_____ c) Red

_____ d) Orange

24. When all three primary colors are present in equal proportions, the resulting color is _____.

25. Black can be made by mixing colors together.

_____ True

_____ False

26. Which of the following is a secondary color?

_____ a) Red

_____ b) Yellow

_____ c) Green

_____ d) Blue

27. Complementary colors neutralize each other.

_____ True

_____ False

28. The stylist should use which of the following colors to neutralize orange?

_____ a) Yellow

_____ b) Violet

_____ c) Blue

_____ d) Green

29. Name the four warm tones that can look lighter than their actual levels.

a) _____

b) _____

c) _____

d) _____

30. _____ refers to the strength of a color.

TYPES OF HAIRCOLOR

31. Identify the two categories of haircoloring products:

a) _____

b) _____

32. Which of the following is a use of demipermanent color?

_____ a) Add subtle results

_____ b) Blend gray hair

_____ c) Create bright changes

_____ d) All answers are correct.

33. Give the roles of an alkalizing ingredient.

a) _____

_____

b) _____

c) _____

34. The pigments in temporary color penetrate the cuticle layer.

_____ True

_____ False

35. Traditional semipermanent haircolor lasts _____ to _____ weeks.

36. Why are demipermanent haircolor products able to deposit without lifting?

_____

_____

_____

37. Permanent haircoloring products are regarded as the best products for covering gray hair.

_____ True

_____ False

38. Natural and metallic haircolors are known as _____ colors.

39. Henna is usually available only in what tones? _____

_____

40. Metallic haircolors have been marketed to women.

_____ True

_____ False

41. A(n) _____ is an oxidizing agent that, when mixed with an oxidation haircolor, supplies the necessary oxygen gas to develop the color molecules and create a change in natural hair color.

42. What volume hydrogen peroxide should you use with high-lift colors?

_____ a) 10

_____ b) 20

_____ c) 30

_____ d) 40

43. List the objectives of hair lighteners.

a) _____

b) _____

c) _____

d) _____

e) _____

44. During the process of decolorizing, natural hair can go through as many as _____ stages.

45. How are toners used? _____

_____

_____

CONSULTATION

46. A haircolor consultation is the most critical part of the color service.

_____ True

_____ False

47. Give some examples of leading questions to ask during the consultation.

a) _____

b) _____

c) _____

d) _____

48. Medications can affect hair color.

_____ True

_____ False

49. What is the purpose of the release statement? _____

_____

_____

_____

_____

HAIRCOLOR FORMULATION

50. List the four basic questions you should always ask when formulating a haircolor.

a) _____

b) _____

c) _____

d) _____

51. Permanent color is applied by what two methods?

a) _____

b) _____

52. A patch test must be given _____ to _____ hours before the application of any aniline haircolor.

53. List the main portions of the pre-service procedure.

a) _____

b) _____

c) _____

d) _____

54. What are the main portions of the post-service procedure?

a) _____

b) _____

c) _____

55. Give the procedure for performing a patch test.

a) _____

_____

b) _____

c) _____

d) _____

_____

e) _____

f) _____

_____

g) _____

HAIRCOLOR APPLICATIONS

56. The strand test is performed before the client is prepared for the coloring service.

_____ True

_____ False

57. Name the materials, implements, and supplies needed for temporary haircolor application.

a) _____

b) _____

c) _____

d) _____

e) _____

f) _____

g) _____

h) _____

i) _____

58. Semipermanent colors only deposit color.

_____ True

_____ False

59. The application procedure for demipermanent haircolor is similar to that of a traditional semipermanent color.

_____ True

_____ False

60. In a(n) _____ application, hair is colored for the first time.

61. Outline the procedure for permanent single-process retouch with a glaze.

a) _____

b) _____

c) _____

d) _____

e) _____

_____

f) _____

_____

g) _____

h) _____

62. What is the purpose of double-process high-lift coloring. _____

_____

_____

63. When lightening virgin hair, lightener should be applied _____ inch(es) (cm) from the scalp.

USING LIGHTENERS

64. Colorists can choose from what three forms of lightener?

a) _____

b) _____

c) _____

65. Name the features and benefits of cream lighteners.

a) _____

b) _____

c) _____

_____

_____

_____

66. _____ are powdered persulfate salts added to haircolor to increase its lightening ability.

67. Discuss the use of powdered off-the-scalp lighteners. _____

_____

_____

_____

_____

68. Why is a preliminary strand test performed? _____

_____

_____

69. Compare the procedure for a lightener retouch with that for lightening virgin hair.

_____

_____

USING TONERS

70. Toners require a double-process application.

_____ True

_____ False

71. Detail the procedure for toner application.

a) _____

b) _____

c) _____

d) _____

e) _____

f) _____

g) _____

_____

SPECIAL EFFECTS HAIRCOLORING

72. _____, also known as lowlighting, is the technique of coloring strands of hair darker than the natural color.

73. What are the three most common methods for achieving highlights?

a) _____

b) _____

c) _____

74. In the procedure for special effects haircoloring with foil, the hair is divided into _____ sections.

75. The _____ technique, also known as the free-form technique, involves painting a lightener (usually powdered off-the-scalp lightener) directly onto clean, styled hair.

76. When are highlighting shampoos used? _____

_____

_____

SPECIAL CHALLENGES IN HAIRCOLOR/CORRECTIVE SOLUTIONS

77. Name the factors that can cause yellowed hair.

a) _____

b) _____

c) _____

d) _____

78. For gray hair, formulations from Level _____ will provide better coverage and can be used to create pastel and blond tones if desired.

79. For hair that is 30 to 50 percent gray, the semipermanent/demipermanent color formulation should be:

_____ a) One level lighter than the desired level

_____ b) Two levels lighter than the desired level

_____ c) Equal parts one and two levels lighter

_____ d) Equal parts desired and one level lighter

80. Give tips for achieving gray coverage.

a) _____

b) _____

c) _____

d) _____

e) _____

f) _____

g) _____

81. _____ is the process of treating gray or very resistant hair to allow for better penetration of color.

82. Give rules for effective color correction.

a) _____

b) _____

c) _____

d) _____

e) _____

f) _____

g) _____

83. List the characteristics of damaged hair.

a) _____

b) _____

c) _____

d) _____

e) _____

f) _____

g) _____

84. _____ fillers are used to recondition damaged, overly porous hair and equalize porosity so that the hair accepts the color evenly from strand to strand and from scalp to ends, while _____ fillers equalize porosity and deposit color in one application to provide a uniform contributing pigment on prelightened hair.

85. Yellow blond hair can be corrected to a natural blond by adding what two colors?

   a) _____

   b) _____

86. Fading is uncommon with color-treated red hair.

   _____ True

   _____ False

87. List haircolor tips for redheads.

   a) _____

   b) _____

   c) _____

   _____

   d) _____

   _____

   e) _____

   _____

   _____

88. What are some haircolor tips for blonds?

   a) _____

   _____

   b) _____

   _____

   c) _____

   d) _____

   _____

   e) _____

   _____

   _____

   _____

   _____

89. What is the solution for hair with a green cast? _____

_____

_____

_____

90. What should the stylist do if the overall hair color is too dark? _____

_____

_____

_____

_____

_____

91. Provide the steps for restoring blond hair to its natural color.

a) _____

_____

_____

_____

_____

_____

_____

b) _____

_____

_____

_____

_____

c) _____

_____

_____

_____

_____

_____

_____

HAIRCOLORING SAFETY PRECAUTIONS

92. List haircoloring safety precautions.

a) _____

_____

b) _____

c) _____

d) _____

e) _____

f) _____

_____

g) _____

h) _____

i) _____

j) _____

k) _____

l) _____

m) _____

n) _____

o) _____

22 Hair Removal

Date: _____

Rating: _____

Text Pages: 685–707

POINT TO PONDER:

"Chance favors the prepared mind."—**Louis Pasteur**

1. Hair removal is one of the fasting growing services in the salon and spa business.

   _____ True

   _____ False

2. _____ is a waxing technique that requires the removal of all hair from the front and the back of the bikini area.

3. Many men are now requesting hair removal services.

   _____ True

   _____ False

4. Men most often request hair removal for which of the following areas?

   _____ a) Nape of the neck

   _____ b) Chest

   _____ c) Back

   _____ d) All answers are correct.

5. The most common form of hair removal in salons and spas is _____.

6. _____, also known as _____, refers to the growth of an unusual amount of hair on parts of the body normally bearing only downy hair, such as the faces of women or the backs of men.

7. Name the two major categories of hair removal.

   a) _____

   b) _____

WHY STUDY HAIR REMOVAL?

8. In your own words, explain why cosmetologists should study and thoroughly understand hair removal. _____

_____

_____

_____

_____

_____

_____

CLIENT CONSULTATION

4. Similar to an intake form, a(n) _____ is a questionnaire that discloses all medications, both topical and oral, along with any known skin disorders or allergies that might affect treatment.

5. List some medications that may render a client unsuited to hair removal services.

a) _____

b) _____

c) _____

d) _____

e) _____

6. How often should clients complete release forms for hair removal services?

_____ a) Every visit

_____ b) Every other visit

_____ c) Every year

_____ d) Once at initial visit

CONTRAINDICATIONS FOR HAIR REMOVAL

7. Waxing or hair removal should not be performed on clients who:

a) _____

b) _____

c) _____

d) _____

e) _____

f) _____

g) _____

h) _____

_____

i) _____

j) _____

k) _____

8. Facial waxing should not be performed on clients with any of the following conditions:

a) _____

b) _____

c) _____

_____

d) _____

e) _____

_____

f) _____

g) _____

PERMANENT HAIR REMOVAL

9. Match each of the following types of permanent hair removal with its definition.

_____ Electrolysis

a) Technique that uses intense light to destroy the growth cells of the hair follicles

_____ Photoepilation

b) Method in which a beam pulses on the skin, impairing hair growth

_____ Laser hair removal

c) Removal by means of an electric current that destroys the growth cells of hair

10. Who can perform electrolysis? _____

_____

11. Who can perform photoepilation? _____

_____

12. Clinical studies have shown that photoepilation can provide _____ to _____ percent clearance of hair in _____ weeks.

13. Laser hair removal is most effective when used on follicles in the _____ or _____ phase.

14. What type of hair responds best to laser treatment? _____

_____

15. Is laser hair removal permanent? _____

_____

16. Who can perform laser hair removal? _____

_____

_____

TEMPORARY HAIR REMOVAL

17. Name the methods of temporary hair removal.

a) _____

b) _____

c) _____

d) _____

e) _____

f) _____

18. _____ is the most common form of temporary hair removal, particularly of men's facial hair.

19. During shaving, _____ can help reduce irritation.

20. Shaving causes hair to grow thicker and stronger.

_____ True

_____ False

21. _____ is commonly used to shape the eyebrows and remove undesirable hairs from around the mouth and chin.

22. List the steps in the pre-service procedure for preparing a facial room.

a. _____

_____

b. _____

c. _____

d. _____

_____

_____

e. _____

f. _____

g. _____

h. _____

_____

_____

_____

_____

i. _____

j. _____

_____

_____

_____

22. Give the steps in the procedure to follow at the end of the day with respect to the facial room.

a) _____

_____

b) _____

_____

c) _____

_____

d) _____

e) _____

_____

_____

f) _____

_____

g) _____

h) _____

i) _____

_____

j) _____

k) _____

_____

_____

_____

_____

23. The natural arch of the eyebrow follows the _____, or the curved line of the eye socket.

24. Explain how to determine the best shape for an eyebrow. _____

_____

_____

_____

_____

_____

_____

25. A(n) _____ is a substance, usually a caustic alkali preparation, used to temporarily remove superfluous hair by dissolving it at the skin surface level.

26. What happens when a depilatory is applied? _____

_____

27. It is a good idea to patch test a depilatory before a first treatment.

_____ True

_____ False

28. Which of the following is *not* appropriate for temporary hair removal from the arms?

_____ a) Waxing

_____ b) Tweezing

_____ c) Depilatories

_____ d) All answers are correct.

29. A(n) _____ removes hair from the bottom of the follicle.

30. Wax is a commonly used epilator.

_____ True

_____ False

31. What makes cold wax different from hot wax? _____

_____

32. The time between waxings is generally _____ to _____ weeks.

33. Wax may be applied to various parts of the face and body, such as the _____, _____, _____, _____, _____, and _____.

34. For a waxing service, hair should be at least _____-inch(es) (cm) long but no longer than _____ inch(es) (cm).

35. Removing _____ or _____ hair may cause the skin to temporarily feel less soft.

36. Before beginning a wax treatment, be sure the client completes a(n) _____ form and signs a(n) _____ form.

37. Why should disposable gloves be worn during waxing? _____

_____

38. List the implements and materials needed for an eyebrow waxing procedure.

a) _____

b) _____

c) _____

d) _____

e) _____

f) _____

g) _____

h) _____

i) _____

j) _____

k) _____

l) _____

39. Explain how to apply wax in the body waxing procedure. _____

_____

_____

_____

_____

39. _____ is a temporary hair removal method in which cotton thread is twisted and rolled along the surface of the skin, entwining the hair in the thread and lifting it from the follicle.

40. Sugaring produces the same results as hot or cold wax.

_____ True

_____ False

41. After sugaring, residue can be dissolved with _____.

Date: _____

Rating: _____

Text Pages: 708–755

POINT TO PONDER:

"To get what you've never had, you must do what you've never done."—**Unknown**

1. Facial treatments can be very relaxing and offer many improvements to the _____ of the skin.

2. Proper skin care can make oily skin look _____, dry skin look and feel more _____, and aging skin look _____

   _____.

WHY STUDY FACIALS?

3. In your own words, explain why cosmetologists should study and thoroughly understand facials. _____

   _____

   _____

   _____

   _____

   _____

   _____

   _____

   _____

SKIN ANALYSIS AND CONSULTATION

4. Discuss the importance of skin analysis. _____

   _____

   _____

5. The opportunity to ask clients questions about their health and skin care history and to advise them about appropriate home-care products and treatments comes during the _____.

6. What is the main purpose of the health screening form? _____

_____

_____

7. A(n) _____ is a condition that requires avoiding certain treatment procedures or products to prevent undesirable side effects.

8. Name the main contraindications to look for.

a) _____

_____

b) _____

c) _____

d) _____

e) _____

f) _____

g) _____

h) _____

i) _____

j) _____

9. Clients with obvious skin abnormalities or other signs of possible skin abnormalities should be referred to a physician for treatment.

_____ True

_____ False

10. What information is obtained via the health screening form?

a) _____

b) _____

c) _____

d) _____

e) _____

f) _____

11. Describe the information the treatment record should provide. _____

_____

_____

_____

_____

_____

12. Cosmetologists should avoid wearing jewelry on the hands or arms while administering facial treatments because _____

_____.

DETERMINING SKIN TYPE

13. _____ is determined by how oily or dry the skin is.

14. Skin type can be permanently changed by treatment.

_____ True

_____ False

15. The amount of sebum produced by the _____ determines the size of the pores and is _____.

16. Obvious pores indicate _____ skin, while lack of pores indicates _____ or _____ skin.

17. The term *alipidic* means _____ and describes skin that produces too little sebum.

18. Normal skin is very unusual.

_____ True

_____ False

19. Which of the following skin types has comedones, clogged pores, or obvious pores in the center of the face?

_____ a) Combination oily

_____ b) Acne

_____ c) Combination dry

_____ d) Oily

20. Oily skin produces too much sebum and will have _____ and may appear to be _____.

21. Describe open comedones: _____

_____

22. Define closed comedones. _____

_____

_____

23. Why is acne considered a skin type? _____

_____

24. Acne bacteria are anaerobic, which means _____

_____.

25. Skin conditions are generally treatable.

_____ True

_____ False

26. Describe dehydration: _____

_____

27. List some causes of dehydration.

a) _____

b) _____

c) _____

28. How is dehydrated skin treated? _____

_____

29. Describe hyperpigmentation: _____

30. How is hyperpigmentation treated? _____

_____

_____

31. Explain how to identify sensitive skin. _____

_____

32. What should you avoid when treating sensitive skin? _____

_____

_____

33. _____ is a chronic hereditary disorder that can be indicated by constant or frequent facial blushing.

34. _____ are distended or dilated surface blood vessels, while _____ are areas of skin with distended capillaries and diffuse redness.

35. Describe aging skin:_____

_____

36. How is aging skin treated? _____

37. Describe sun-damaged skin: _____

_____

_____

_____

_____

_____

_____

SKIN CARE PRODUCTS

38. Name the two types of cleanser.

a) _____

b) _____

39. Toners, also known as _____ or _____, are lotions that help rebalance the pH and remove remnants of cleanser from the skin.

40. Exfoliants can improve the appearance of wrinkles, aging, and hyperpigmentation.

_____ True

_____ False

41. _____ are peeling creams, also called roll-off masks, that are rubbed off of the skin.

42. Discuss the use of alpha hydroxy acids. _____

_____

_____

_____

_____

_____

43. Compare the two basic types of keratolytic enzyme peels. _____

_____

_____

_____

_____

_____

_____

44. Name some ways in which exfoliation improves the skin's appearance.

a) _____

b) _____

c) _____

d) _____

e) _____

f) _____

g) _____

45. Oily skin does not need much emollient.

_____ True

_____ False

46. Shielding the skin from sun exposure is probably the most important habit to benefit the skin.

_____ True

_____ False

47. _____ are individual doses of serum, sealed in small vials.

48. Cream masks do not dry on the skin and are often used to moisturize dry skin.

_____ True

_____ False

49. Discuss the preparation and application of modelage masks. _____

_____

_____

_____

_____

_____

_____

_____

50. Describe the use of gauze for mask application: _____

_____

_____

_____

_____

_____

_____

_____

CLIENT CONSULTATION

51. All facial treatments should begin with a(n) _____.

52. What information should the client consultation card contain?

a) _____

b) _____

c) _____

d) _____

_____

e) _____

f) _____

_____

g) _____

h) _____

i) _____

_____

53. During the consultation, it is important to perform a thorough _____ _____ before cleansing.

FACIAL MASSAGE

54. _____ is the manual or mechanical manipulation of the body by rubbing, gently pinching, kneading, tapping, and using other movements to increase metabolism and circulation, to promote absorption, and to relieve pain.

55. In facial massage, the direction of movement is always _____

_____.

56. Describe effleurage: _____

_____

57. Pressure is a key component of effleurage.

_____ True

_____ False

58. Describe pétrissage: _____

_____

59. Fulling is used mainly for massaging the _____.

60. List and describe the variations of friction.

a) _____

_____

_____

b) _____

_____

c) _____

_____

_____

_____

61. Tapotement is the most stimulating form of massage.

_____ True

_____ False

62. Name the body parts on which hacking is used.

a) _____

b) _____

c) _____

63. Vibration should be applied at the _____ of massage.

64. Every muscle has a _____ point, which is a point on the skin that covers the muscle where pressure or stimulation will cause contraction of that muscle.

65. _____ is achieved through light but firm, slow, rhythmic movements or very slow, light, hand vibrations over the motor points for a short time.

66. Name the benefits of proper face and scalp massage.

a) _____

b) _____

c) _____

d) _____

e) _____

f) _____

g) _____

67. How does a cosmetologist perform linear movement over the forehead?

_____

_____

_____

68. What facial movement does the accompanying figure illustrate? _____

_____

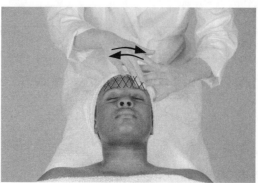

69. Explain how to perform the light tapping movement. _____

_____

_____

70. Describe how to perform the chest and back movement. _____

_____

_____

FACIAL EQUIPMENT

71. A facial _____ heats water and produces a stream of warm steam that can be focused on the client's face or other areas of skin.

72. _____ brushes are used for back treatment, while _____ brushes are used for the face.

ELECTROTHERAPY AND LIGHT THERAPY

73. Identify the contraindications of electrotherapy. _____

_____

_____

_____

74. Galvanic machines have two positive electrodes called a(n) _____, which has a red plug and cord, and a negative electrode, called a(n) _____, which has a black plug and cord.

75. Desincrustation is very helpful when treating oily areas with multiple comedones and most acne-prone skin.

_____ True

_____ False

76. _____ is the process of using galvanic current to enable water-soluble products that contain ions to penetrate the skin.

77. Microcurrent is best known for helping to tone the skin, producing a lifting effect for aging skin that lacks elasticity.

_____ a) True

_____ b) False

78. Compare direct application and indirect massage. _____

_____

_____

_____

_____

79. Discuss the use of light-emitting diode (LED) treatment in cosmetology.

_____

_____

_____

_____

_____

_____

80. _____ is a type of mechanical exfoliation that involves shooting aluminum oxide or other crystals at the skin with a handheld device that exfoliates dead cells.

FACIAL TREATMENTS

81. Facial treatments fall into what two categories?

a) _____

b) _____

82. A preservative treatment is meant to _____

_____

_____ .

83. A corrective treatment is meant to _____

_____ .

84. What are the guidelines for performing a facial treatment?

a) _____

b) _____

_____

c) _____

d) _____

_____

e) _____

f) _____

g) _____

85. List the main tasks of the pre-service procedure.

a) _____

b) _____

c) _____

86. Name the basic sections of the post-service procedure.

a) _____

b) _____

87. What equipment is optional for a basic facial?

a) _____

b) _____

c) _____

88. How should the client prepare for a basic facial? _____

_____

89. Where should the client change prior to the facial? _____

_____

90. Give the procedure for draping the client's hair for a basic facial.

a) _____

_____

_____

b) _____

_____

_____

c) _____

_____

_____

91. Discuss how to steam a client's face for a basic facial. _____

_____

_____

_____

_____

92. What is the proper procedure for applying a treatment mask during a basic facial?

a. _____

_____

b. _____

_____

c. _____

_____

d. _____

93. How is the treatment mask removed during a basic facial? _____

_____

94. After the treatment mask is removed during a basic facial, what should be applied? _____

_____

95. List the procedure for a dry-skin facial.

a) _____

b) _____

c) _____

_____

d) _____

_____

_____

_____

e) _____

f) _____

g) _____

h) _____

_____

i) _____

j) _____

k) _____

_____

_____

_____

l) _____

m) _____

_____

n) _____

o) _____

_____

p) _____

q) _____

_____

_____

_____

_____

_____

_____

_____

r) _____

_____

s) _____

_____

_____

t) _____

_____

u) _____

_____

v) _____

w) _____

x) _____

_____

96. In addition to the items needed for a basic facial, what items are needed for a facial on oily skin with comedones?

a) _____

b) _____

c) _____

d) _____

97. When treating acne-prone skin, disposable gloves should be worn throughout the treatment.

_____ True

_____ False

98. Minor problem skin and oily skin responds poorly to facial treatments.

_____ True

_____ False

99. How can cosmetologists help clients with acne-prone skin?

_____

_____

_____

100. Acne-prone skin should not be massaged.

_____ True

_____ False

101. After extraction is complete in a facial for acne-prone and problem skin, what steps must the cosmetologist complete?

a) _____

_____

_____

_____

b) _____

_____

_____

c) _____

d) _____

_____

_____

_____

_____

e) _____

_____

f) _____

g) _____

_____

h) _____

_____

102. Home care is probably the most important factor in a successful skin care program.

_____ True

_____ False

AROMATHERAPY

103. The therapeutic use of plant aromas for beauty and health treatment is known as _____.

104. Cosmetologists are qualified to perform healing treatments with aromatherapy.

_____ True

_____ False

CHAPTER 24 Facial Makeup

Date: _____

Rating: _____

Text Pages: 756–790

POINT TO PONDER:

"May it be said, when the sun sets on your life, you made a difference."—**Unknown**

1. Makeup is a part of cosmetology that is very interesting and can produce _____ and _____ changes in the appearance.

WHY STUDY FACIAL MAKEUP?

2. In your own words, explain why cosmetologists should study and thoroughly understand facial makeup. _____

_____

_____

_____

_____

_____

_____

_____

_____

COSMETICS FOR FACIAL MAKEUP

3. List the forms of foundation.

a) _____

b) _____

c) _____

4. A(n) _____ is applied to the skin before foundation to cancel out and help disguise skin discoloration.

5. Skin primers are applied after any colored foundation.

_____ True

_____ False

6. Most liquid and cream forms of makeup contain a base mixture of _____ spreading agents that contain a significant amount of _____ and various color agents called _____.

7. _____ foundations often quickly produce a(n) _____ finish, meaning they dry to become nonshiny.

8. _____ foundations are usually intended for dry skin types and tend to produce a shiny appearance.

9. Cosmetic products that cause the formation of clogged pores are called _____, which means that they produce comedones.

10. Explain how to choose the correct foundation color. _____

_____

_____

_____

_____

_____.

11. A(n) _____ is an obvious line where foundation starts or stops.

12. Contrast how the different types of foundation are applied. _____

_____

_____

_____

_____

13. _____ are a thick, heavy type of foundation used to hide dark eye circles, dark splotches, and other imperfections.

14. A concealer may be worn alone, without foundation.

_____ True

_____ False

15. Explain how to apply concealer. _____

_____

_____

_____

_____

16. What is the purpose of face powder? _____

_____

_____

17. Some face powders that contain little color are called _____.

18. Describe how loose face powder is applied: _____

_____

_____

_____

_____

_____

19. _____ blush is used immediately after the foundation to blend color into the foundation, while _____ blush is used after both the foundation and powder have been applied.

20. Powder blush should be applied in a circle on the apple of the cheek, beyond the corner of the eye, or inward between the cheekbone and the nose.

_____ True

_____ False

21. Lip color must never be applied directly from the container unless the container belongs to the client.

_____ True

_____ False

22. After lip color has been removed from the container, how is it applied?

_____

_____

_____

23. Eye shadow comes in what forms?

a) _____

b) _____

c) _____

d) _____

24. Cosmetologists should avoid matching eye shadow to eye color because

_____ .

25. A(n) _____ shade of eye color makes the natural color of the iris appear lighter, while a lighter shade makes the iris appear _____ .

26. A(n) _____ color is generally a medium tone that is close to a client's skin tone. A(n) _____ color is a color, in any finish, that is deeper and darker than the client's skin tone.

27. Most clients prefer eyeliner that is the same color as the _____ for a more natural look. More dramatic colors may be chosen depending on _____ .

28. How are eyebrow pencils used? _____

_____

_____

29. Eyebrow pencils should be sanitized before each use.

_____ True

_____ False

30. The most popular mascara colors are shades of _____ and _____, which enhance the natural lashes by making them appear thicker and longer.

31. Mascara may be used on all the lashes from the _____ .

32. When applying mascara, it is okay to double dip the wand.

_____ True

_____ False

33. When using an eyelash curler, when should you curl the lashes? _____

_____

34. _____ is a heavy makeup used for theatrical purposes. _____ _____, also known as pancake makeup, is a heavy-coverage makeup pressed into a compact and applied to the face with a moistened cosmetic sponge.

35. Match each of the following makeup implements with its use.

_____ 1. Powder brush   a) Remove excess facial hair

_____ 2. Blush brush   b) Apply shadow to the eyebrows or shadow liner to the eyes

_____ 3. Concealer brush   c) Apply powder cheek color

_____ 4. Lip brush   d) Diffuse and blend shadow

_____ 5. Eye shadow brushes   e) Lift and upward curl the upper lashes

_____ 6. Eyeliner brush   f) Apply concealer around the eyes or over blemishes

_____ 7. Angle brush   g) Remove excess mascara from lashes or comb brows into place

_____ 8. Lash and brow brush   h) Apply powder and blend edges of color

_____ 9. Tweezers   i) Apply liquid liner or shadow to the eyes

_____ 10. Eyelash curler   j) Apply concealer or lip color

36. Discuss the procedures for cleaning makeup brushes. _____

_____

_____

_____

_____

_____

_____

_____

_____

_____

_____

37. List the disposable implements used for a makeup service.

a) _____

b) _____

c) _____

d) _____

e) _____

f) _____

g) _____

h) _____

i) _____

MAKEUP COLOR THEORY

38. Define primary, secondary, and tertiary colors. _____

_____

_____

_____

_____

_____

_____

_____

_____

_____

39. Identify the three main factors to consider when choosing colors for a client.

a) _____

b) _____

c) _____

40. _____ colors are the range from yellow and gold through the oranges, red-oranges, most reds, and even some yellow-greens. _____ colors suggest coolness and are dominated by blues, greens, violets, and blue-reds.

41. Pale peach is a warm color for which of the following skin colors?

_____ a) Light

_____ b) Medium

_____ c) Dark

_____ d) All answers are correct.

42. A neutral skin tone contains equal elements of warm and cool, no matter how light or dark the skin is.

_____ True

_____ False

43. If skin color is light, use _____ colors for a soft, natural look; _____ colors will create a more dramatic look.

44. If skin color is medium, medium tones will create a(n) _____ look. Light or dark tones will provide more _____ and will appear bolder.

45. If skin color is dark, dark tones will be more _____. Medium to medium-light or bright tones will be _____.

46. Matching eye shadow with eye color is the best way to enhance the eye area.

_____ True

_____ False

47. What are the steps for color selection?

a) _____

b) _____

c) _____

d) _____

e) _____

f) _____

_____

g) _____

_____

h) _____

48. _____ is the complementary color to blue. Red is the complementary color to _____. _____ eyes are neutral and can wear any color.

49. The cosmetologist should coordinate cheek and lip makeup in the same color family as eye makeup.

_____ True

_____ False

50. The cosmetologist should mix warm and cool colors on a face.

_____ True

_____ False

51. _____ color needs to be taken into account when determining eye makeup color.

52. Blue is a cool color for which of the following hair colors?

_____ a) Blonde

_____ b) Red

_____ c) Brown

_____ d) Black

BASIC PROFESSIONAL MAKEUP APPLICATION

53. What is the cosmetologist's role in a makeup consultation? _____

_____

_____

54. Give guidelines for maintaining the consultation area. _____

_____

_____

_____

_____

_____

_____

55. Artificial light is best for makeup consultations.

_____ True

_____ False

56. What is the role of a client instruction sheet? _____

_____

_____

_____

57. Give the steps to complete to prepare for a client as part of the pre-service procedure.

a) _____

_____

_____

b) _____

_____

_____

c) _____

_____

d) _____

_____

_____

e) _____

58. Outline the end-of-the-day portion of the post-service procedure.

a) _____

_____

b) _____

_____

_____

c) _____

_____

d) _____

e) _____

_____

_____

f) _____

_____

g) _____

h) _____

i) _____

_____

j) _____

k) _____

_____

_____

_____

_____

59. To test the color of foundation as part of basic professional makeup application, blend the foundation on the client's _____.

60. Once you have selected its color, where should you place the foundation?

_____

_____

61. Where should you begin to blend foundation when performing a basic professional makeup application? _____

_____

_____

62. How do you apply concealer as part of basic professional makeup application?

_____

_____

_____

63. If a powder foundation is being used as part of a basic professional makeup application, the concealer must be applied _____ the foundation.

64. After applying concealer as part of a basic professional makeup application, apply _____.

65. What should you use to apply powder during a basic professional makeup application, and how should you apply it? _____

_____

_____

_____

_____

66. Why would you use a moistened cosmetic sponge over finished makeup?

_____

67. When performing a basic professional makeup application, select a(n) _____ color in a medium tone and then, beginning at the _____, apply lightly and blend _____ with a brush or disposable applicator.

68. Describe how to apply eyeliner as part of a basic professional makeup application: _____

_____

_____

_____

69. Where should mascara be applied during a basic professional makeup application? _____

_____

70. How should you determine where to put blush when performing a basic professional makeup application? _____

_____

_____

71. Explain how to apply lip liner as part of the basic professional makeup application procedure. _____

_____

_____

_____

_____

_____

_____

_____

_____

_____

_____

_____

_____

SPECIAL-OCCASION MAKEUP

72. Outline the procedure for creating striking contour eyes.

a) _____

_____

b) _____

_____

c) _____

_____

d) _____

_____

e) _____

_____

f) _____

_____

_____

g) _____

73. Give the steps to creating dramatic smoky eyes.

a) _____

b) _____

c) _____

_____

_____

_____

d) _____

e) _____

_____

f) _____

g) _____

74. Give some tips for creating a special occasion look for the cheeks.

a) _____

_____

_____

b) _____

_____

75. Give some tips for creating a special occasion look for lips.

a) _____

b) _____

_____

c) _____

CORRECTIVE MAKEUP

76. Shadowing emphasizes a feature, while highlighting minimizes it.

_____ True

_____ False

77. The basic rule of makeup application is to _____ the client's attractive features, while _____ features that are less appealing.

78. The face is divided into three equal _____ sections. The first third is measured from the _____. The second third is measured from the _____. The last third is measured from the _____.

79. The ideal oval face is approximately _____ as wide as it is long.

80. The distance between the eyes is the width of _____.

81. The round face is usually broader in proportion to its length than the oval face.

_____ True

_____ False

82. The _____ face is composed of comparatively straight lines with a wide forehead and square jawline.

83. A jaw that is wider than the forehead characterizes the _____ _____face.

84. The _____ or heart-shaped face has a wide forehead and narrow, pointed chin.

85. The _____ face has a narrow forehead with the greatest width across the cheekbones.

86. The _____ face has greater length in proportion to its width than the square or round face.

87. For a _____ forehead, a lighter foundation lends a broader appearance between the brows and hairline.

88. For a _____ forehead, darker foundation over the prominent area gives an illusion of fullness to the rest of the face and minimizes the bulging forehead.

89. For a _____ nose, apply a darker foundation on the nose and a lighter foundation on the cheeks at the sides of the nose.

90. If the nostrils are wide, apply a(n) _____ foundation to both sides of the nostrils. For a broad nose, use a(n) _____ foundation on the sides of the nose and nostrils.

91. For a(n) _____ chin and receding nose, shadow the chin with a darker foundation and highlight the nose with a lighter foundation.

92. For a(n) _____ chin, highlight the chin by using a lighter foundation than the one used on the face.

93. For a(n) _____ chin, use a darker foundation on the sagging portion and use a natural skin tone foundation on the face.

94. To correct a(n) _____ jawline, apply a darker shade of foundation over the heavy area of the jaw, starting at the temples.

95. To correct a(n) _____ jawline, highlight by using a lighter foundation shade.

96. For a(n) _____ face, apply a darker shade of foundation over the prominent part of the jawline.

97. For a _____ face and a _____ neck, use a darker foundation on the neck than the one used on the face.

98. For a(n) _____ neck, apply a lighter shade of foundation on the neck than the one used on the face.

99. _____ eyes can be lengthened by extending the shadow beyond the outer corner of the eyes.

100. _____ eyes are closer together than the length of one eye.

101. For eyes that are too close together, lightly apply shadow up from the _____.

102. _____ eyes can be minimized by blending the shadow carefully over the prominent part of the upper lid, carrying it lightly toward the eyebrow.

103. For _____ eyes, shadow evenly and lightly across the lid from the edge of the eyelash line to the small crease in the eye socket.

104. For _____ eyes, apply the shadow on the upper inner side of the eyelid, toward the nose, and blend carefully.

105. For _____ eyes, use bright, light, reflective colors. Use the lightest color in the crease and use a light-to-medium color sparingly on the lid and brow bone.

106. For _____ under eyes apply concealer over the area, blending and smoothing it into the surrounding area.

107. The eyebrow is the _____ for the eye, and overgrown eyebrows can cast a(n) _____ on the brow bone or between the two eyebrows.

108. _____ eyebrows can make the face look puffy or protruding or may give the eyes a surprised look.

109. Ideally, the eyebrow begins _____.

110. The second line to determine the ideal eyebrow shape is drawn at an angle from the _____ to the outer corner of the eye.

111. The third line of the ideal eyebrow shape is vertical, from the _____

_____.

112. What should you do if the eyebrow arch is too high? _____

_____

_____

113. People with low foreheads should wear a _____, which gives more height to a very low forehead.

114. If a person has _____ eyes, extend the eyebrow lines to the inside corners of the eyes.

115. If a person has _____ eyes, widen the distance between the eyebrows and slightly extend them outward.

116. If a person has a round face, arch the brows _____ to make the face appear narrower.

117. If a person has a long face, making the eyebrows almost _____ can create the illusion of a shorter face.

118. If a person has a square face, the face will appear more oval if there is a(n) _____ arch on the ends of the eyebrows.

119. _____ are lash lengtheners that contain fibers to make lashes look longer and fuller.

120. Lips are usually proportioned so that the curves or peaks of the upper lip fall directly in line with the nostrils.

_____ True

_____ False

121. What can you do for a client who has ruddy skin? _____

_____

122. What can you do for a client who has sallow skin? _____

_____

_____

ARTIFICIAL EYELASHES

123. _____, also known as strip lashes, are eyelash hairs on a strip that are applied with adhesive to the natural lash line.

124. List the implements and materials needed to apply band lashes.

a) _____

b) _____

c) _____

d) _____

e) _____

f) _____

g) _____

h) _____

i) _____

j) _____

k) _____

l) _____

m) _____

n) _____

o) _____

p) _____

q) _____

r) _____

125. In band lash application, why is lower lash application optional? _____

_____

25 Manicuring

Date: _____

Rating: _____

Text Pages: 791–841

POINT TO PONDER:

"If you don't have a dream, how you gonna have a dream come true?"—**"Happy Talk" from Rodgers and Hammerstein's South Pacific**

1. The list of services cosmetologists are legally allowed to perform in their specialties in their states is known as the _____

2. A Scope of Practice may state the services cosmetologists cannot legally perform.

   _____ True

   _____ False

3. If a client sustains damage while a cosmetologist is performing an illegal service, the cosmetologist is not liable.

   _____ True

   _____ False

WHY STUDY MANICURING?

4. In your own words, explain why cosmetologists should study and thoroughly understand manicuring. _____

   _____

   _____

   _____

   _____

   _____

NAIL TECHNOLOGY TOOLS

5. Professional cosmetologists must learn to work with the tools required for nail services and know all _____, _____, and _____ procedures as defined in state regulations.

6. Name the four types of nail technology tools cosmetologists incorporate into their services.

a) _____

b) _____

c) _____

d) _____

7. _____ includes all nonimplement, permanent tools used to perform nail services.

8. List the equipment needed to perform nail services.

a) _____

b) _____

c) _____

d) _____

e) _____

f) _____

g) _____

h) _____

i) _____

j) _____

k) _____

l) _____

m) _____

n) _____

o) _____

9. A manicuring table can vary in length, but it is usually _____ to _____ inches (meters) long.

10. The adjustable lamp attached to a manicuring table should be 40 to 60 watts or fluorescent.

_____ True

_____ False

11. The cosmetologist's chair should be selected for what features?

_____

_____

12. The Occupational Safety and Health Act (OSHA) defines _____
_____ as "specialized clothing or equipment worn by an employee
for protection against a hazard."

13. Define the term bloodborne pathogen (BBP). _____

_____

_____

14. Explain how to remove the gloves worn during nail services. _____

_____

_____

_____

_____

15. When a client receives a manicure and a pedicure, the cosmetologist needs only
one set of gloves.

_____ True

_____ False

16. Name the steps for handling an exposure incident during a manicure.

a) _____

_____

b) _____

_____

c) _____

d) _____

e) _____

_____

_____

f) _____

_____

_____

_____

g) _____

_____

17. How is the fingerbowl used in nail service? _____

_____

18. The federal Environmental Protection Agency (EPA) requires total immersion of implements during disinfection.

_____ True

_____ False

19. The warmth of electric hand/foot mitts is designed to _____

_____, _____, and _____

_____.

20. _____, a petroleum by-product, has excellent sealing properties to hold moisture in the skin.

21. _____ or _____ implements are generally stainless steel because they must be properly cleaned and disinfected after use on one client and before use on another.

22. _____ or _____ implements cannot be reused because they cannot be cleaned and disinfected; they must be thrown away after one use.

23. Match each of the following implements with its use in nail care.

_____ 1. Wooden pusher

_____ 2. Metal pusher

_____ 3. Nail brush

_____ 4. Nippers

_____ 5. Tweezers

a) Trim away dead skin around nails

b) Shorten the nail's free edge quickly and efficiently

c) Remove products from containers

d) Remove cuticle tissue from the nail plate or clean under the nail's free edge

e) Scrub implements clean before disinfection

_____ 6. Nail clippers

f) Lift small bits of debris from the nail plate and remove implements from disinfectant solution

_____ 7. Plastic or metal spatula

g) Apply nail oils, nail polish, or nail treatments

_____ 8. Two- or three-way buffer

h) Create a beautiful shine on nails

_____ 9. Application brush

i) Gently scrape cuticle tissue from the natural nail plate

24. Lower-grit abrasives, which are less than _____ grit, are aggressive, while fine-grit abrasives, in the category of _____ and higher grit, are designed for buffing, polishing, and removing very fine scratches.

PROFESSIONAL COSMETIC PRODUCTS

25. Why are liquid soaps preferred professional cosmetic products? _____

_____

_____

_____

26. _____ are used to dissolve and remove nail polish.

27. _____ polish works more quickly and is a better solvent than _____ removers, which are preferred when removing nail polish from nail enhancements.

28. What are nail creams, lotions, and oils designed to do? _____

_____

_____

29. Discuss the use of cuticle removers in nail care. _____

_____

_____

30. Excessive exposure of the eponychium to cuticle removers can cause _____

_____.

31. What is nail bleach? _____

_____

_____

32. What are the alternate names for the colored coatings applied to the natural nail plate?

a) _____

b) _____

c) _____

d) _____

33. _____ is a generic term describing any type of solvent-based, colored film applied to the nail plate for the purpose of adding color or special visual effects.

34. Why is it important to use base coats on nail enhancements? _____

_____

_____

35. Nail hardeners can be applied before the base coat or after as top coat.

_____ True

_____ False

36. List some basic types of nail hardeners.

a) _____

b) _____

c) _____

37. By law, home-care products must be accompanied by usage directions and cautions or written instructions.

_____ True

_____ False

38. Discuss the use of top coats in cosmetology. _____

_____

39. Contrast hand creams and lotions. _____

_____

_____

_____

_____

_____

40. _____ provide valuable safe-handling information about products, as well as first aid and proper storage information.

41. Experts say that as much as _____ percent of skin damage is caused by exposure to the sun.

THE BASIC MANICURE

42. Before leaving school, cosmetologists should work to get the basic manicure procedure to _____ minutes at the most, including polishing.

43. Give the two choices for providing clean brushes for cosmetology services.

a) _____

b) _____

_____

44. Outline the process for cleaning and disinfecting implements as part of the pre-service procedure. _____

_____

_____

_____

_____

_____

_____

45. List the steps in the post-service procedure.

a) _____

_____

_____

b) _____

_____

_____

_____

c) _____

_____

_____

d) _____

_____

e) _____

_____

46. Detail the procedure for proper hand washing.

a) _____

_____

b) _____

_____

_____

_____

c) _____

_____

_____

_____

_____

d) _____

_____

e) _____

_____

_____

f) _____

_____

g) _____

_____

47. According to the CDC, hand sanitizers can replace hand washing in most circumstances.

_____ True

_____ False

48. During the manicure consultation, what qualities should the cosmetologist consider?

a) _____

b) _____

c) _____

49. Explain how to shape nails as part of the basic manicure procedure.

_____

_____

_____

_____

_____

_____

_____

_____

_____

50. What does the accompanying figure depict? _____

_____

_____

51. Discuss what the cosmetologist should do when performing a basic manicure on a client with yellow nails. _____

_____

_____

_____

_____

52. Why should a cosmetologist exercise caution when buffing the nail plate during a basic manicure? _____

_____

_____

53. List the five basic nail shapes women most often prefer.

a) _____

b) _____

c) _____

d) _____

e) _____

54. List the four coats of a successful nail polish application.

a) _____

b) _____

c) _____

d) _____

55. Discuss the procedure for applying colored nail polish. _____

_____

_____

_____

_____

_____

_____

_____

_____

_____

_____

_____

56. Applying nail polish layer by layer improves adhesion and staying power.

_____ True

_____ False

57. When applying iridescent or frosted polish, the strokes should be _____ to the sidewalls of the nails to avoid shadow lines in the polish.

A MAN'S MANICURE SERVICE

58. A man's manicure is executed using the basic manicure procedure, though you omit the _____.

59. Square nails are the most common choice for male clients.

_____ True

_____ False

60. Why must the cosmetologist prepare a man's nails for polish carefully?

_____

_____

61. Explain how a salon can effectively market nail services to men. _____

_____

_____

_____

_____

_____

_____

_____

_____

_____

_____

_____

MASSAGE

62. _____ is the manipulation of the soft tissues of the body.

63. The cosmetologist should always have one hand on the client's arm or hand during massage procedures.

_____ True

_____ False

64. Identify the massage movements that are usually combined to complete a massage.

a) _____

b) _____

c) _____

d) _____

e) _____

65. _____ is a succession of strokes in which the hands glide over an area of the body with varying degrees of pressure or contact.

66. What events are essential after a massage? _____

_____

_____

67. Describe the position the cosmetologist should assume before performing a hand and arm massage. _____

_____

_____

_____

68. Hand and/or arm massage is contraindicated for clients with _____

_____ .

69. Discuss how to massage the forearm as part of the hand and arm massage procedure. _____

_____

_____

_____

_____

_____

_____

_____

70. What does the accompanying figure depict? _____

_____

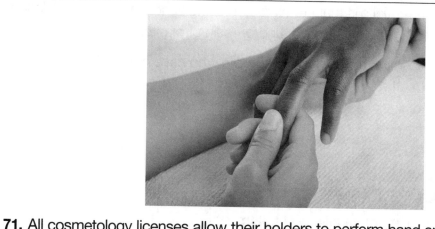

71. All cosmetology licenses allow their holders to perform hand and foot massages.

_____ True

_____ False

SPA MANICURES

72. Spa manicures require more advanced techniques than basic manicures.

_____ True

_____ False

73. All spa manicures include some form of _____ not only for polishing and smoothing the skin but also for enhancing penetration of professional products.

74. Some products for spa manicures are chemical free.

_____ True

_____ False

75. Identify the additional techniques that may be incorporated into a spa manicure.

a) _____

b) _____

c) _____

AROMATHERAPY

76. The practice of _____ involves the use of highly concentrated, non-oily, and volatile essential oils that are extracted using various forms of distillation from seeds, bark, roots, leaves, wood, and/or resin of plants.

77. Blended oils are safe and easy to use by people who have not studied aromatherapy in depth.

_____ True

_____ False

PARAFFIN WAX TREATMENT

78. Explain the basic intent of paraffin wax treatments. _____

_____

_____

_____

79. Special heating units melt solid wax into a gel-like liquid and maintain it at a temperature generally between _____ and _____ degrees Fahrenheit.

80. Name the advantages of performing a paraffin wax treatment before beginning a manicure.

a) _____

_____

b) _____

81. Detail the procedure for performing a paraffin wax treatment during a manicure.

a) _____

b) _____

c) _____

d) _____

_____

e) _____

_____

f) _____

g) _____

_____

_____

_____

h) _____

CHAPTER 26 Pedicuring

Date: _____

Rating: _____

Text Pages: 842–871

POINT TO PONDER:

"Whoever is happy will make others happy too."—**Anne Frank**

1. A(n) _____, a cosmetic service performed on the feet by a licensed cosmetologist or nail technician, can include exfoliating the skin, reducing calluses, and trimming, shaping, and polishing the toenails.

2. Pedicures are merely manicures on the feet.

   _____ True

   _____ False

3. Pedicures can cause more damage to clients than manicures.

   _____ True

   _____ False

4. Give some reasons why pedicures are beneficial.

   1. _____

   2. _____

   3. _____

WHY STUDY PEDICURING?

5. In your own words, explain why cosmetologists should study and thoroughly understand pedicuring. _____

   _____

   _____

   _____

   _____

PEDICURE TOOLS

6. Name the four types of nail technology tools the cosmetologist will use.

a. _____

b. _____

c. _____

d. _____

7. Some permanent equipment for pedicures differs from that for manicures.

_____ True

_____ False

8. Which of the following pieces of pedicure equipment is considered optional?

_____ a. Paraffin bath

_____ b. Pedicure footrest

_____ c. Pedicure cart

_____ d. Foot bath

9. Give some examples of pedicure foot baths in increasing order of sophistication.

_____

_____

_____

_____

_____

_____

_____

_____

_____

_____

_____

10. Contrast electric foot mitts with terry cloth mitts. _____

_____

_____

_____

_____

_____

_____

_____

11. List some pedicure-specific implements.

a. _____

b. _____

c. _____

d. _____

e. _____

f. _____

12. Identify the materials unique to pedicuring, as well as their uses.

a. _____

b. _____

_____

c. _____

_____

13. Name the professional products that are unique to pedicuring.

a. _____

b. _____

c. _____

d. _____

e. _____

14. _____ are products containing gentle soaps, moisturizers, and other additives that are used in the pedicure bath to cleanse and soften the skin.

15. Exfoliating scrubs are usually _____-based lotions that contain a(n) _____ as the exfoliating agent.

16. What are some popular ingredients in masks? _____

_____

17. Callus softeners are applied directly to clients' heels and over pressure-point calluses.

_____ True

_____ False

ABOUT PEDICURES

18. Give some guidelines for choosing pedicure products. _____

_____

_____

_____

_____

_____

_____

_____

19. Discuss the benefit of short pedicure services. _____

_____

_____

_____

20. Why should female clients avoid shaving their legs for the 48 hours preceding a pedicure? _____

_____

_____

_____

21. The basic pedicure in most salons includes a leg massage.

_____ True

_____ False

22. Discuss the concept of the series pedicure, and give an example. _____

_____

_____

23. What are the three parts of a pedicure?

a) _____

b) _____

c) _____

24. Name the basic tasks performed during the pre-service procedure.

a. _____

b. _____

c. _____

25. What should the cosmetologist do during the post-service procedure?

a. _____

b. _____

26. List the steps for a pedicure pre-service.

a) _____

b) _____

c) _____

d) _____

e) _____

f) _____

g) _____

27. During the client consultation, you should:

a) _____

b) _____

c) _____

d) _____

_____

28. If infection or inflammation is present, what should you do? _____

_____

29. When using a manufacturer's product line, it is recommended that you follow
their _____.

30. How should you make your client feel during the service? _____

_____

31. When handling the foot, be _____ , but _____ .

32. Describe how to grasp the foot when performing a pedicure: _____

_____

33. What does grasping the foot during a pedicure accomplish?

a) _____

b) _____

_____

34. Name the five basic steps involved in the actual pedicure service.

a) _____

b) _____

c) _____

d) _____

e) _____

35. During the actual pedicure procedure, what should you discuss with your client?

_____

_____

36. On which side of the client should the basic pedicure start, and why? _____

_____

_____

_____

37. In the basic pedicure, the big toe is usually the most challenging to trim.

_____ True

_____ False

38. Describe how to use a foot rasp during the basic pedicure procedure:

_____

_____

_____

_____

39. Explain how to use lotion or oil during a foot and leg massage. _____

_____

_____

_____

_____

_____

_____

40. The bottom of the foot is the only place a friction movement is performed in pedicure services.

_____ True

_____ False

41. What is the role of feathering in foot and leg massage? _____

_____

_____

_____

42. Describe the subject of the accompanying figure: _____

_____

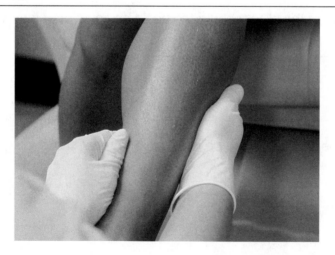

43. Older people need less regular foot care than younger people.

_____ True

_____ False

44. For an elderly client receiving pedicure services, a microscopic opening, or _____ , can be fatal.

45. According to Merriam-Webster's Dictionary, the term _____ is defined as "a method of manipulation of the body by rubbing, pinching, kneading, tapping."

46. Massage given during manicures and pedicures focuses on therapy.

_____ True

_____ False

47. Give a brief overview of reflexology. _____

_____

_____

_____

_____

48. List the two reasons professional, hands-on training is essential in reflexology.

a. _____

_____

b. _____

_____

49. Pedicures can threaten the health and well-being of the cosmetologists who perform them.

_____ True

_____ False

DISINFECTION

50. Outline the procedure for disinfecting whirlpool foot spas and air-jet basins after every client.

a. _____

b. _____

_____

_____

c. _____

d. _____

_____

_____

e. _____

51. When disinfecting pipe-less foot spas, list the steps that should be completed at the end of every day.

a. _____

_____

_____

_____

b. _____

c. _____

_____

_____

d. _____

52. Give some examples of non-whirlpool foot basins or tubs.

a. _____

b. _____

c. _____

d. _____

e. _____

27 Nail Tips and Wraps

Date: _____

Rating: _____

Text Pages: 872–895

POINT TO PONDER:

"There are no shortcuts to any place worth going."—**Beverly Sills**

WHY STUDY NAIL TIPS AND WRAPS?

1. In your own words, explain why cosmetologists should study and thoroughly understand nail tips and nail wraps._____

_____

_____

_____

_____

_____

_____

_____

_____

_____

NAIL TIPS

2. Nail tips are plastic, pre-molded nails shaped from a tough polymer made from _____ plastic.

3. Tips are combined with a(n) _____, a layer of any kind of nail enhancement product that is applied over the natural nail and tip application for added strength.

4. In addition to basic materials, what implements are needed on the manicuring table?

   a) _____

   b) _____

   c) _____

d) _____

e) _____

5. Fingernail clippers should be used to cut tips.

_____ True

_____ False

6. Define the roles of the well and the position stop. _____

_____

_____

_____

7. The bonding agent used to secure the nail tip to the natural nail is called the

_____.

8. Cosmetologists and their clients should always wear eye protection when using and handling nail tip adhesives.

_____ True

_____ False

9. Give the steps in the cleaning and disinfecting portion of the pre-service procedure.

a) _____

_____

_____

b) _____

_____

_____

_____

c) _____

_____

_____

_____

_____

d) _____

_____

_____

_____

e) _____

_____

f) _____

g) _____

_____

10. Outline the steps in the post-service procedure.

a) _____

_____

b) _____

_____

_____

c) _____

_____

_____

_____

d) _____

_____

e) _____

_____

f) _____

_____

g) _____

_____

11. Explain the proper way to apply adhesive during nail tip application. _____

_____

_____

_____

_____

_____

_____

12. Detail the steps in nail tip removal.

a) _____

_____

b) _____

_____

_____

_____

c) _____

_____

d) _____

_____

NAIL WRAPS

13. Any method of securing a layer of fabric or paper on and around the nail tip to ensure its strength and durability is called a(n) _____.

14. Wrap resins are made from _____, a specialized acrylic monomer that has excellent adhesion to the natural nail plate and polymerizes in seconds.

15. Fabric wraps are the most popular type of nail wrap because of their durability.

_____ True

_____ False

16. Compare silk wraps and linen wraps. _____

_____

_____

_____

_____

_____

_____

_____

17. Why are paper wraps considered a temporary service? _____

_____

_____

_____

18. A(n) _____, also known as an activator, acts as the dryer that speeds the hardening process of the wrap resin or adhesive overlay.

19. Name the implements and materials needed for nail wrap application.

a) _____

b) _____

c) _____

d) _____

e) _____

f) _____

g) _____

20. Describe the method known as Dip Powder and Adhesive Enhancements.

_____

_____

_____

_____

_____

NAIL WRAP MAINTENANCE, REPAIR, AND REMOVAL

21. What two goals does nail maintenance accomplish?

a) _____

_____

b) _____

_____

22. Outline the steps to 2-week fabric wrap maintenance.

a) _____

_____

b) _____

c) _____

d) _____

e) _____

_____

_____

_____

f) _____

_____

g) _____

_____

_____

h) _____

_____

i) _____

j) _____

_____

k) _____

l) _____

m) _____

_____

_____

n) _____

23. Explain how to buff the nail during the procedure for 4-week fabric wrap
maintenance. _____

_____

_____

_____

_____

_____

_____

24. What is a stress strip? _____

_____

_____

_____

25. Discuss the proper procedure for removing fabric nail wraps. _____

_____

_____

_____

_____

_____

CHAPTER 28 Monomer Liquid and Polymer Powder Nail Enhancements

Date: _____

Rating: _____

Text Pages: 896–923

POINT TO PONDER:

"Success seems to be connected with action. Successful people keep moving. They make mistakes, but they don't quit."—**Conrad Hilton**

1. Nail enhancements based on mixing liquids and powders are commonly called _____ nails.

2. Monomer liquid and polymer powder nail enhancement products are based on _____.

WHY STUDY MONOMER LIQUID AND POLYMER POWDER NAIL ENHANCEMENTS?

3. In your own words, explain why cosmetologists should study and thoroughly understand monomer liquid and polymer powder nail enhancements.

_____

_____

_____

_____

_____

_____

_____

_____

MONOMER LIQUID AND POLYMER POWDER NAIL ENHANCEMENTS

4. Monomer liquid and polymer powder nail enhancements, also called
_____, are created by combining _____ liquid, a chemical
liquid, and _____ powder, a powder in white, clear, pink, and many other
colors, to form the nail enhancement.

5. _____ means one and _____ stands for units, so a(n) _____ is
one unit called a molecule. _____ means many, so _____ means a
substance formed by combining many small molecules into very long, chain-like
structures.

6. List the three basic ways monomer liquid and polymer powder products can be
applied.

a) _____

b) _____

c) _____

7. Give the steps in the basic table setup portion of the pre-service procedure.

a) _____

_____

b) _____

_____

_____

_____

c) _____

_____

_____

_____

_____

_____

_____

d) _____

_____

_____

e) _____

_____

f) _____

_____

_____

_____

_____

g) _____

_____

h) _____

_____

_____

_____

_____

_____

_____

8. Detail the steps in the post-service procedure.

a) _____

_____

b) _____

_____

_____

_____

c) _____

_____

_____

d) _____

_____

e) _____

_____

f) _____

_____

g) _____

_____

9. In addition to the basic materials on the manicuring table, name the supplies needed for the One-Color Monomer Liquid and Polymer Powder Nail Enhancements over Nail Tips or Natural Nails procedure.

a) _____

b) _____

c) _____

d) _____

e) _____

f) _____

g) _____

10. A(n) _____ brush is the best brush to apply one-color monomer liquid and polymer powder nail enhancements over nail tips or natural nails.

11. List the three versions of monomer liquid used to apply one-color monomer liquid and polymer powder nail enhancements over nail tips or natural nails.

a) _____

b) _____

c) _____

12. Describe what occurs during the chemical reaction called polymerization.

_____

_____

_____

13. _____, substances that speed chemical reactions between monomer liquid and polymer powder, are added to monomer liquid and used to control the set or curing time. _____ are substances that start chain reactions in which monomer molecules begin permanently linking into long polymer chains.

14. Explain why it is important to use the polymer powder designed for a specific monomer liquid. _____

_____

_____

MONOMER LIQUID AND POLYMER POWDER NAIL ENHANCEMENT SUPPLIES

15. The amount of monomer liquid and polymer powder used to create a bead is called the _____.

16. Compare dry, medium, and wet mix ratios. _____

_____

_____

_____

_____

17. In general, medium beads are the ideal mix ratio for working with monomer liquids and polymer powders.

_____ True

_____ False

18. The color of polymer powder depends on the nail enhancement method.

_____ True

_____ False

19. Explain the use of nail dehydrators. _____

_____

_____

20. Acid-based nail primers are used most often today.

_____ True

_____ False

21. High-quality hand sanitizers can replace hand washing in many cases.

_____ True

_____ False

22. Outline the procedure for using nonacid and acid-free nail primers. _____

_____

_____

_____

_____

_____

_____

_____

_____

_____

23. Choose a(n) _____ grit for smoothing and a(n) _____ buffer for final buffing.

24. _____ are placed under the free edge of the nail to extend nail enhancements beyond the fingertip.

25. In the procedure for two-color monomer liquid and polymer powder nail enhancements using forms, how many dappen dishes are used, and for what purpose? _____

_____

_____

26. Describe the appropriate containers for monomer liquid and polymer powder.

_____

_____

_____

_____

_____

_____

27. The best way to dispose of small amounts of monomer liquid is to mix them with small amounts of the powder designed to cure them.

_____ True

_____ False

28. Explain why sable-hair brushes are best for monomer liquid and polymer powder nail enhancements. _____

_____

_____

29. Dust masks are worn to provide vapor protection.

_____ True

_____ False

30. For many salon-related applications, gloves made of nitrile polymer powder work best.

_____ True

_____ False

31. Explain how to store monomer liquid and polymer powder products. _____

_____

_____

_____

MONOMER LIQUID AND POLYMER POWDER NAIL ENHANCEMENT MAINTENANCE, CRACK REPAIR, AND REMOVAL

32. What is the preferred maintenance schedule for monomer liquid and polymer powder nail enhancements? _____

_____

33. Give the steps in the one-color monomer liquid and polymer powder maintenance procedure.

a) _____

b) _____

_____

_____

c) _____

_____

_____

_____

d) _____

_____

e) _____

_____

_____

f) _____

g) _____

h) _____

i) _____

_____

_____

j) _____

k) _____

_____

l) _____

_____

_____

_____

m) _____

_____

n) _____

_____

_____

_____

o) _____

_____

_____

p) _____

q) _____

r) _____

s) _____

t) _____

34. List the steps for crack repair for monomer liquid and polymer powder nail enhancements.

a) _____

b) _____

_____

c) _____

d) _____

e) _____

f) _____

g) _____

_____

_____

h) _____

_____

i) _____

_____

j) _____

k) _____

l) _____

_____

m) _____

n) _____

o) _____

p) _____

35. The _____ of the nail, also known as arch, is the area of the nail that has all the strength.

36. The stress area is the area on the side of the nail plate that grows free of its attachment to the nail fold and where the extension leaves the natural nail.

_____ True

_____ False

37. Discuss the nail extension underside. _____

_____

_____

_____

_____

_____

_____

38. Name the steps in the procedure for monomer liquid and polymer powder nail enhancement removal.

a) _____

_____

_____

b) _____

_____

_____

c) _____

_____

_____

_____

_____

_____

_____

_____

_____

d) _____

e) _____

f) _____

ODORLESS MONOMER LIQUID AND POLYMER POWDER PRODUCTS

39. Odorless monomer liquid and polymer powder products have a slight odor.

_____ True

_____ False

40. Define the inhibition layer of odorless products, and explain how to remove it.

_____

_____

_____

_____

_____

_____

_____

COLORED POLYMER POWDER PRODUCTS

41. Polymer powders are now available in a wide range of colors that mimic almost every shade available in nail polish.

_____ True

_____ False

29 UV Gels

Date: _____

Rating: _____

Text Pages: 924–954

POINT TO PONDER:

"People never improve unless they look to some standard or example higher and better than themselves."—**Tyron Edwards**

1. A(n) _____ is a type of nail enhancement product that hardens when exposed to a UV light source.

WHY STUDY UV GELS?

2. In your own words, explain why cosmetologists should study and thoroughly understand UV gels.

_____

_____

_____

_____

_____

_____

_____

UV GELS

3. Nail enhancements based on UV curing are very similar to methacrylates.

_____ True

_____ False

4. UV gel enhancements rely on ingredients from a chemical family called _____.

5. Like wraps and monomer liquid and polymer powder nail enhancements, UV gels can contain _____ liquids, but they rely mostly on a related form called a(n) _____ .

6. The term *oligo* means which of the following?

   _____ a) One

   _____ b) Many

   _____ c) Few

   _____ d) Outside

7. Discuss the concept of an oligomer. _____

   _____

   _____

8. Oligomers are between solid and liquid.

   _____ True

   _____ False

9. Traditionally, UV gels rely on a special type of acrylate called a(n) _____ acrylate, while new UV gel systems use _____ .

10. The term _____ refers to the type of starting material used to create the most common UV gel resins.

11. The chemical family of urethanes is known for durability.

   _____ True

   _____ False

12. A chemical called a(n) _____ causes UV gel resins to react when exposed to the UV light recommended for the gel.

13. UV gels typically use a powder that is cured to a solid material when exposed to a UV light source.

   _____ True

   _____ False

14. After the nail plate is properly prepared, each layer of product that is applied requires exposure to UV light to _____, or harden.

15. Identify the different types of UV gels.

a) _____

b) _____

c) _____

d) _____

16. Describe the one-color method for applying UV gels. _____

_____

_____

_____

17. List the steps to the table setup portion of the pre-service procedure.

a) _____

b) _____

_____

_____

_____

c) _____

_____

_____

_____

_____

_____

_____

d) _____

_____

_____

e) _____

_____

f) _____

_____

g) _____

_____

_____

h) _____

_____

i) _____

_____

_____

_____

18. Explain how, as part of the post-service procedure, to schedule the next appointment and thank a client.

a) _____

_____

_____

b) _____

_____

c) _____

_____

19. Name the implements and materials for the one-color method for applying UV gel on tips or natural nails.

a) _____

b) _____

c) _____

d) _____

e) _____

f) _____

g) _____

h) _____

i) _____

20. Discuss how to apply the first layer of UV gel to the fingernail surface using the one-color method. _____

_____

_____

_____

_____

_____

_____

21. Detail the two-color method for applying UV gel to tips or natural nails.

a) _____

b) _____

c) _____

d) _____

e) _____

f) _____

g) _____

h) _____

i) _____

_____

_____

_____

_____

_____

j) _____

_____

_____

k) _____

_____

_____

_____

l) _____

m) _____

_____

n) _____

_____

_____

_____

o) _____

p) _____

_____

q) _____

_____

_____

_____

_____

r) _____

s) _____

_____

t) _____

u) _____

v) _____

w) _____

x) _____

y) _____

z) _____

aa) _____

bb) _____

cc) _____

_____

22. _____ are used to increase adhesion to the natural nail plate, similar to a monomer liquid and polymer powder primer.

23. A bonding product that is not cured in an ultraviolet light unit is less effective than one cured in a UV light unit.

_____ True

_____ False

24. Which of the following type of UV gels is used to enhance the thickness of the overlay while providing a smoother surface?

_____ a) UV gel polish

_____ b) Pigmented UV gel

_____ c) UV gloss gel

_____ d) UV self-leveling gel

25. UV _____ gels are very helpful when repairing a break or crack in a client's enhancement.

26. A(n) _____ layer is a tacky surface left on the nail after a UV gel has cured.

27. Opacity is the concentration of colored pigment in a gel.

_____ True

_____ False

UV GEL SUPPLIES

28. In addition to the supplies in the basic manicuring setup, what items are needed for UV gel enhancement?

a) _____

b) _____

c) _____

d) _____

e) _____

f) _____

g) _____

h) _____

i) _____

j) _____

WHEN TO USE UV GELS

29. When should clients use UV gels? _____

_____

_____

30. Explain how to refine the surface contour when applying UV gel over forms.

_____

_____

_____

_____

31. Discuss the special considerations when applying the third UV gel (sealer or finisher UV gel) as part of applying UV gel over monomer liquid and polymer powder nail enhancements. _____

_____

_____

_____

_____

_____

CHOOSING THE PROPER UV GEL

32. Give some guidelines for choosing the proper UV gel.

a) _____

_____

b) _____

_____

c) _____

_____

UV LIGHT UNITS AND LAMPS

33. Differentiate between UV lamps and UV light units. _____

_____

_____

_____

_____

34. Unit wattage is the measure of how much electricity a lamp consumes.

_____ True

_____ False

35. If a UV gel product is exposed to ceiling or table lamps while in its container, what may occur? _____

_____

_____

36. Why is it important to use the UV lamp that was designed for the UV gel product being used? _____

_____

_____

37. How often should UV bulbs be changed?

_____ a) Monthly

_____ b) Once annually

_____ c) Two or three times annually

_____ d) Every 1 to 3 years

38. Give some potential results of failing to regularly change UV lamps.

a) _____

b) _____

c) _____

39. The most common UV lamp on the market is _____-watt.

_____ a) 4

_____ b) 6

_____ c) 7

_____ d) 9

40. A light unit has as much to do with proper curing of UV gel as the lamp.

_____ True

_____ False

UV GEL POLISH

41. Name some advantages of UV gel polishes.

a) _____

b) _____

42. Describe how to remove a UV gel polish. _____

_____

_____

_____

_____

UV GEL MAINTENANCE AND REMOVAL

43. Explain how to begin/prepare for UV gel maintenance. _____

_____

_____

_____

_____

_____

_____

_____

44. Outline the procedure for UV gel maintenance.

a) _____

b) _____

c) _____

d) _____

_____

_____

e) _____

f) _____

g) _____

h) _____

_____

_____

_____

_____

i) _____

j) _____

_____

k) _____

l) _____

m) _____

_____

_____

_____

_____

n) _____

o) _____

p) _____

q) _____

r) _____

s) _____

t) _____

u) _____

_____

v) _____

45. Give the two types of gel and their methods of removal.

a) _____

_____

b) _____

_____

46. List the steps for removing hard UV gel.

a) _____

b) _____

_____

c) _____

_____

_____

d) _____

_____

_____

47. Outline the procedure for removing soft UV gel.

a) _____

b) _____

c) _____

_____

_____

d) _____

_____

e) _____

_____

f) _____

_____

_____

g) _____

_____

CHAPTER 30 Seeking Employment

See Milady Standard Cosmetology Theory Workbook.

CHAPTER 31 On the Job

See Milady Standard Cosmetology Theory Workbook.

CHAPTER 32 The Salon Business

See Milady Standard Cosmetology Theory Workbook.